Diagnostic and treatment algorithms in neurology

Gulsum Duchshanova
Sergei Chumakov
Elvira Zulfikarova

Diagnostic and treatment algorithms in neurology

LAP LAMBERT Academic Publishing RU

Imprint

Any brand names and product names mentioned in this book are subject to trademark, brand or patent protection and are trademarks or registered trademarks of their respective holders. The use of brand names, product names, common names, trade names, product descriptions etc. even without a particular marking in this work is in no way to be construed to mean that such names may be regarded as unrestricted in respect of trademark and brand protection legislation and could thus be used by anyone.

Cover image: www.ingimage.com

Publisher:
LAP LAMBERT Academic Publishing
is a trademark of
International Book Market Service Ltd., member of OmniScriptum Publishing Group
17 Meldrum Street, Beau Bassin 71504, Mauritius

Printed at: see last page
ISBN: 978-613-9-84408-1

Copyright © Gulsum Duchshanova, Sergei Chumakov, Elvira Zulfikarova
Copyright © 2018 International Book Market Service Ltd., member of OmniScriptum Publishing Group
All rights reserved. Beau Bassin 2018

Diagnostic and treatment algorithms in neurology

2018

UDK 616.8 (075.8)
BBK 56.1
Ch-D.862
ISBN 978-613-9-84408-1

The manual was prepared by the Doctor of Medicine, Professor. Duchshanova G.A. - Head of the Chair of Neurology, Psychiatry and Psychology of the South Kazakhstan State Medical University, associate Professors Zulfikarova E.T., Chumakov S.A.

"Diagnostic and treatment algorithms in neurology"

The manual is intended for students of medical universities, interns, residents, magistrates, doctors of students of F of AP, neurologists, neurosurgeons, psychiatrists, general practitioners, resuscitators.

Reviewers:

Doctor of Medical Sciences, Professor Baidaulet I.O.

Candidate of Medical Sciences, associate professor Zholymbekova L.D.

Thanks to the authors:

I.Salmyrza for their participation in the translation

2018

INTRODUCTION

The task of neurological diagnosis, as in other clinical specialties, is the knowledge of the internal nature of the disease, which largely determines the role of diagnostics in the broad activity of a neurologist. The detailed characterization of the symptoms, their analysis, being a necessary part of the diagnostic process, makes it possible to isolate any particulars, details from the general picture of the disease.

Syndrome in neurology is a combination of symptoms, linked together pathogenetically or topically. The syndromological approach to the analysis and evaluation of pathological symptoms is important not only for the subsequent stage of recognizing the nature of the disease, but also for substantiating pathogenetic therapy.

Algorithms, charts and tables allow the doctor to quickly navigate in the diagnostic search and diagnosis, give the opportunity to follow the most rational path, get rid of unnecessary work, warn against errors. Mastering the main stages of the diagnostic process provides the doctor with guidance in a wide variety of complex situations. Improving the diagnosis of neurological diseases is mainly through the development of more complex, subtle and reliable methods of research. But this is not the only way. Significant improvement and acceleration of diagnostics can be achieved by optimizing clinical thinking.

It is important for the practical doctor to achieve maximum diagnostic results on the basis of a minimum set of examinations. This is to the maximum extent the method of syndromic algorithm (the algorithm is a prescription about step-by-step execution in a certain sequence of elementary operations for solving problems of this class). To establish the diagnosis, it takes less time and requires significantly fewer different medical studies than conventional diagnostic practice.

The clinical thinking of the neurologist is based on a consistent knowledge of the neurological symptoms, then integrating them into syndromes, with the transition to nosological forms of disease in the future through a differential diagnosis.

It should not be forgotten that the direct methods of neurological examination of the patient retain their leading significance and at the present time, when methods of laboratory, instrumental and neurovisual research have become widespread.

The newest medical technologies alone can not replace the clinical thinking of a doctor. The art of diagnostics consists in the rational use of modern technical capabilities, skilfully interpreting the obtained laboratory, instrumental data.

Diseases of the peripheral nervous system
Classification

I. Vertebrogenic lesions
1. Cervical level.
1.1. Reflex syndromes. 1.1.1. Cervicalgia.
1.1.2. Cervicocranialgia (posterior cervical sympathetic syndrome, and others.).
1.1.3. Cervicobrahialgia with muscular-tonic or vegetative-vascular or neurodystrophic manifestations.
1.2. Radicular syndromes
1.2.1. Discogenic (vertebrogenic) lesion ("radiculitis") of roots (specify which ones).
1.3. Radicular-vascular syndromes (radiculo-ischemia).
2. Thoracic level.
2.1. Reflex syndromes.
2.1.1. Thoracalgia with muscular-tonic or vegetative-visceral, or neurodystrophic manifestations.
2.2. Radicular syndromes.
2.2.1. Discogenic (vertebrogenic) lesion ("radiculitis") of roots (specify which ones).
3. Lumbosacral osteochondrosis.
3.1. Reflex syndromes.
3.1.1. Lumbago (chamber).
3.1.2. Lumbalgia.
3.1.3. Lumbosciatica with muscular-tonic or vegetative-vascular, or neurodystrophic manifestations.
3.2. Radicular syndromes.
3.2.1. Discogenic (vertebrogenic) lesion (radiculitis) of rootlets (indicate which ones, including the horse tail syndrome).
3.3. Radicular-vascular syndromes (radiculo-ischemia).

II. Lesions of nerve roots, nodes, plexuses
1. Meningoradiculitis, radiculitis (cervical, thoracic, lumbosacral).
2. Ralikulogaloglionitis, ganglionitis (spinal sympathetic), truncites.
3. Plexitis.
4. Plexus injuries.
4.1. Shaynoy.
4.2. Upper brachial (Erba-Duchenne palsy).
4.3. Lower humerus (paresis of Dejerine-Clumpke).
4.4. Shoulder (total).

4.5. Lumbosacral (partial or total).

III. Multiple lesions of roots, nerves
1. Infectious-allergic polyradiculoneuritis (Guillain-Barre and other.)
2. Infectious polyneuritis.
3. Polyneuropathies.
3.1. Toxic.
3.1.1. With chronic domestic and industrial intoxications (alcoholic, lead, chlorophosic, and other .)
3.1.2. At toxic infections (diphtheria, botulism).
3.1.3. Medicamentous.
3.1.4. Blastomatous: with cancer of the lungs, stomach, and other.
3.2. Allergic (vaccinal, serum, medicamental, and other.)
3.3. Dysmetabolic: with a deficiency of vitamins, with endocrine diseases - diabetes mellitus, etc., with diseases of the liver, kidneys, and other.)
3.4. Dyscirculatory - with nodular periarteritis, rheumatic and other vasculitis.
3.5. Idiopathic and hereditary forms.

IV. Lesions of individual spinal nerves.
1. Traumatic.
1.1. On the upper extremities: radial, ulnar, median, muscular-cutaneous and other nerves.
1.2. On the lower extremities: femoral, sciatic, fibular, tibial and other nerves.
2. Compression-ischemic (mononeuropathy).
2.1. On the upper limbs.
2.1.1. Carpal tunnel syndromes (involvement of the median nerve in the hand area).
2.1.2. Guillain canal syndrome (involvement of the ulnar nerve in the hand area).
2.1.3. Syndrome of the cubital canal (involvement of the ulnar nerve in the ulnar region).
2.1.4. The defeat of the radial or median nerves in the ulnar region, the defeat of the suprascapular, axillary nerves.
2.2. On the lower limbs: syndrome of the tarsal canal, peroneal nerve, lateral cutaneous nerve of the thigh (infringement under the puertal ligament - parathetic MALALGIA Roth-Bernhardt).
3. Inflammatory (mononeuritis).
V. Lesions of the cranial nerves.
1. Neuralgia of the trigeminal and other cranial nerves.
2. Neuritis, facial nerve neuropathy.
3. Neuritis of other cranial nerves.

4. Prozopalgia.
4.1. Ganglionitis (ganglioneuritis) of the pterygoid, ciliary, ear, submandibular and other nodes.
4.2. Combined and other forms of prozopalgin.
5. Stomatalgia, glossalgia.

In addition to the etiology and localization of the process, it is indicated:

1) the nature of the course (acute, subacute, chronic), and in chronic: progredient, stable (protracted), recurrent often, rarely, recombinant;

2) stage (usually in the case of recurrent flow);

3) the nature and extent of the impairment of the functions: the severity of the pain syndrome (mild, moderate, severe, severe), the localization and extent of motor disorders, the severity of sensitivity disorders, vegetative-vascular or trophic disorders, the frequency and severity of paroxysms, seizures.

Conditional Symbols and Abbreviations

DE-Dyscirculatory encephalopathy
CT-Computed tomography
REG-Rheoecephalogram
USDG-Ultrasound dopplerography
SH-Scale of Hamilton
ZQ- Questoinnaire of Zunga
SQQ- Guestionnaire of Spielberger Hanina
EPE-Experimental-psychological examination
EEG-Electroencephalography
MRI-Madnetic resonance imaging
ICD-International classification of diseeasees
ADSC-Acute disturbance of cerebral circulation
CDCC-Chronic disturbance of cerebral circulation
RHA-Republican hospital of ambulance
BIC-Brigade of intensive care
MP-Medical point
PMP-Paramedic midwife point
MOPC-Medical outpatient clinic
CDH-Central district of hospital
AS-Ambulance station
MHD-Magnetic heart disease
AP-Arterial pressure
PHR-Pressureof Heart rate
TPC-Therapeutic physical culture
THA-Trunk Head Arteries
ECEC-Echo cardiac electrocardiography
SH-Subarachnoid haemorrhage
IH-Intracerebral haemorrhage

CN-Craniocerebral nerves
MSS-Marital Stupor Syrgery
AA-An Ambulatory artery
AH-Ambulance Hospital
ALV-Artifical lung Ventilation
MSEC-Medical and social expert Commission
SA-Sistal and Arterial blood pressure
DBP-Diastolic blood Pressure
TT-Thrombolytic therapy
INR-International normalized ratio
APTT-Activated Partial thromboplastin time
CF-Cerebrospinal fluid

Cervical Irritative Reflex Syndromes

Painful

cervicalgia: intense, tingling, boring or dull pain in the deep sections of the neck. This pain is most pronounced in the mornings, after sleep, intensified by turning the head, coughing, sneezing, laughing.

cervicocranyalgia: pain localized in the neck and occipital region.

cervicobrahialgia: pain in the neck is combined with aching pain in the deep sections of the shoulder and forearm (vegetative, sclerotomous).

Muscular-tonic syndromes

syndrome of the lower oblique muscle of the head: constant, lumbent pain in the cervico-occipital region, paresthesia in the occiput, hyperalgesia in the zone of innervation of the large occipital nerve, painful palpation of the points of attachment of the lower oblique muscle of the head, increased pain in the cervical-occipital region when the head rotates to the healthy side.

syndrome of the muscle that lifts the scapula (scapula-rib syndrome): pain (aching, cerebral, in the neck in the upper - inner corner of the scapula, in the shoulder, radiating to the shoulder joint, shoulder, or lateral surface of the chest).

neurodystrophic syndrome: osteochondrosis + impaired function of the shoulder joint due to pain and contracture

Differential diagnostic differences of neurological syndromes caused by pathological changes of the spine

The nature of changes in the spine	Clinical signs	Spondylography results	CSF	Blood
Osteochondrosis	Severe pain syndrome. Compression root and vascular syndromes. Vegetative Irritative Syndromes. Expressed static-dynamic violations	Degenerative changes in intervertebral discs (decrease in height, hernia). Horizontally directed growths of osteophytes	Without changes	Without changes
Spondylosis	Asymptomatic flow or moderate pain. Rarely myelopathy. Immobilization of the corresponding spine.	Calcification of the longitudinal ligament of the spine. Bony "beak-shaped" growths along the vertebrae edges followed by fixation of the latter	Without changes	Without changes
Spondylarthrosis	Perhaps a long asymptomatic course. Vegetative, neurodystrophic and vascular syndromes. Radicular compression syndromes and vegetative - irritative syndromes appear only when combined with osteochondrosis. Pain and crunch in the affected parts during movements	Narrowing of joint cracks. Subchondral osteochondrosis. Elongation and deformation of articular processes	Without changes	Changes correspond to changes in arthrosis
Bechterew's disease	In an early stage of pain, the type of lumboschialgia with irradiation into the inguinal region. Pain in large	Defeat of joints of intervertebral arches and sacroiliac joints. In the initial		Increase in ESR to 50-60 mm/h

11

	The most characteristic symptoms	Diseases with which a differential
Tuberculous spondylitis	Non-localized pain in the spine, reducing pain in the prone position. Signs of tuberculous intoxication (subferbrile, increased fatigue, sweating, weight loss, tachycardia). Muscular, radicular pain: myotonic cushion in interblade area. Syndrome of compression of the spinal cord joints, muscles. Kyphosis, kyphoscoliosis of the thoracic region. "Stiffness" of posture. In the late stages of neurologic symptoms are absent, periodic pain may persist stage, fibrosis and calcification of the discs with the formation of ossifying syndesmophytes. The spine looks like a bamboo stick	Caverns in the bodies of the vertebrae. Compression fractures of vertebral bodies. Destruction of discs and the formation of a stain. Ossification of fibrous rings and longitudinal ligaments of the spine in the form of staples and marginal growths. Kyphotic Deformation	Characteristic decrease in the content of sugar in the CSF, pleocytosis, it is possible violation of permeability of the cerebrospinal fluid	Characteristic for tuberculosis intoxication, an increase in ESR, lymphocytosis Protein-cell dissociation
Malignant (primary and metastatic) tumors	Sharp growing pains in the spine, intensifying at night. Instability of the spine	Destruction of the vertebra, sometimes pathological compression. Intactness of intervertebral discs	Protein-cell dissociation

Differential diagnosis of vertebrogenic cervical localization syndromes

Intervertebral openings	Names of the root and symptoms	The most characteristic symptoms of defeat	Diseases with which a differential
C1-2	C2 (big occipital	Paroxysmal sharp pains in the back of the	Painful muscular densities on the side

	syndrome)	neck like neuralgia. Violation of sensitivity on the side of pain. Pain point in the place of the exit of the large occipital nerve under the skin. Possible development of spastic torticollis syndrome	of the lesion are foci of neuro-osteofibrosis. Craniovertebral anomalies. Disorders of the upper vegetative ganglia
C3-4	C3	Unilateral pain in the neck and in the tongue. Sensation of a "lump" making it hard to swallow and breath	Craniovertebral anomalies. Diseases of the larynx. Neurotic phenomena (hysterical "clot")
C4-5	C4(frenkussindrom)	Pain in the area of the forehead, collarbone, hiccough. Atrophy of the back muscles of the neck	Pathological processes in the mediastinum and lungs. Diseases of the gastrointestinal tract, gallbladder
C7-8	C7	Pain in the neck region is irradiated by the outer surface of the forearm in the third finger. Hypesesia in the zone innervated by the affected spine. Weakness and hypotension of the triceps arm muscle. Reduction or absence of an elbow dilatation reflex	Radiation and median damage nerves (tunnel neuropathy). Cervical anomaly (additional rib), leading to ischemia of the neuromuscular bundle
C7	C8	Pain from the neck radiates to the V finger. Hypalgesia in the zone innervated by the affected spine. Decrease or absence of styloradial and supinator reflexes. Possible development of Horner's syndrome	Injury of the ulnar nerve (tunnel neuropathy). Damage of the brachial plexus. Neurovascular syndromes
C3-5	C4-5(C6)	It is difficult to lift and rotate the shoulder outwards. It is impossible to have a hand	Damage to the suprascapal nerve. Muscular-tonic reflex syndromes

C1-4	C1-4 (cervical plexus)	Forced position and restriction of head movements. With a bilateral defeat, the "drooping head". Pain in the head, neck and shoulder. Impaired sensation in the posterior region of the neck, collarbone	The defeat of the anterior horns and roots of the spinal cord in tick-borne encephalitis and other infectious diseases. Syringomyelia
C3-5	C4-6	Pain in the shoulder and scapula. The lag of the scapula from the chest. Unstable hypesthesia in the shoulder and shoulder area	Traumatic injuries of shoulder area
C4-5	C5	Pain in the neck, radiating to the shoulder and the outer edge of the shoulder. Weakness and hypotension of the deltoid muscle. Hypalgesia over the outer surface of the shoulder	Damage to the subclavian nerve. Compression neurovascular neck syndromes
C5-6	C6	Pain in the neck and shoulder area extend to the shoulder and on the outer surface of the shoulder to the first finger. Paresthesia in the distal parts of the same zone. Paresis of the biceps. Absence of flexion elbow reflexes	Damage of the musculocutaneous, median nerves (tunnel neuropathy). Pathological changes in autonomic neck formations, compression musculo- tonic syndromes

(continued from previous: behind your back. Atrophy of muscles in the scapula area. Possible pain in the shoulder joint)

In all cases, vertebrogenic syndromes due to osteochondrosis should be differentiated from tumor lesions such as neurin or meningitis, as well as diseases of the lymph nodes of the neck region.

Painful points

Localization of pain points

- Spines and paravertebral region
- Intercostal areas of the cervical, axillary and peri-chest lines
- An epigastric region to the right of the midline
- Paravertebral area at the level of X-XII thoracic vertebrae (Boa point)
- Point of spinous processes of VIII-IX thoracic vertebrae (Openchovsky Point)
- Outer edge of right rectus abdominis and costal arch
- The lower edge of the costal arch on the right (Ortner point)
- Above the clavicle, between the legs of the sternocleid - mastoid muscle (Mussie's point)

Diseases and pathological conditions

- Osteochondrosis, herniated intervertebral discs, extramedullary tumors, destructive changes in vertebrae
- Lesion of the intercostal nerve, vegetative ganglia at the appropriate level
- Solarium, reflex solyalgies, cholecystitis, gastroduodenitis
- Stomach ulcer, gastroduodenitis
- Cholecystitis
- Liver diseases
- Muscular-tonic syndrome and diseases accompanied by irritation of the diaphragmatic nerve (osteochondrosis, sub-diaphragmatic abscess, cholecystitis, and other.)

Differential and diagnostic signs of lesions of cervical roots and brachial plexus

Etiological and clinical factors	Lesion of the cervical roots: cervico-brachial radiculopathy (with infection)	Damage of the brachial plexus - upper Erb-Duchenne syndrome	Damage of the brachial plexus-lower Dejerine-Clumpke	Edema and Key Syndrome	Paget-Shreter syndrome	Koreshkovo-vegetative syndromes
Etiological factors	Cervical osteochondrosis, microtrauma, neurinoma and other tumors, infectious and allergic processes	Injuries of the shoulder, clavicle or large vessel (aneurysm rupture), compression by a tumor or enlarged lymph nodes	Shoulder dislocation, trauma of the plexus, clavicle and I rib, compression by a tumor or enlarged lymph nodes, pathological processes in the apex of the lung	Nerve bundle compression between the clavicle and I vein, narrowing of the costal or I interostechnical space	Acute occlusion of the subclavian vein, much more often develops in women, angiotropho neurosis in combination with osteochondrosis	The disease begins after 40 years, inflammation, irritation of the recurrent nerve and parasympathetic fibers. Degenerative changes in the spine
Localization and	Acute, prolonged pain	Unstable pain in the	Long aching pain in a	Diffuse pain in the	Moderate pain in the cervico-	Paroxysmal painful pain. Paroxysmal, intensifying pains in

	nature of pain	Factors that increase pain	Reducing muscle strength and limiting the amount of movement
	in the region of the neck, neck with irradiation in the arm, sometimes in the III- Vials Localization and nature of pain	Movement head, especially fast, a symptom of Sperling, coughing, sneezing, bending the neck (sharp)	Slight, mainly due to pain
shoulder area		Sometimes movements in the shoulder joint	The defeat of the proximal muscle group, the inability to raise the arm above the horizontal
number of cases with a causal shade in the area of the wrist		Sometimes movements in shoulder joint and hand	The defeat of the muscles of the hand and forearm. There are no movements in the hand, fingers,
shoulder, extending to the arm		Pain intensifies at night, patients can not sleep on their side working with their arms raised	Moderate weakness when working with raised hands
humeral region, extending throughout the entire arm. A feeling of pressure in the axillary region		Turns of the head, movements in the shoulder joint, physical activity. Stay in the cold	Suddenly growing swelling and difficulty of active movements in the shoulder and elbow
in the hands at night		Exercise stress. Wearing heavy winter clothes. Meteotropic factors	Difficulty in squeezing a hand into a fist in the morning due to pastosity
the neck, shoulder and hand of a burning, burning nature. Neuropsychiatric disorders (asthenodepressive, hypochondriac or dysphoric reactions)		Emotional stress. Meteotropic factors. Pain is worse at night and when you turn your head	Reduction of muscle tone on the affected side

	t in the arm	reduced strength			joints		
Muscle Atrophy	Occasionally - in the shoulder region	Pronounced atrophy of the muscles of the shoulder and forearm joint	Atrophy of the muscles of the hand and forearm	Common but not very pronounced	Absent	Absent	Absent
Protective muscle tension	In the neck area on the side of the lesion. Symmetrical with meninguriculitis	Can be absent	Absent	Absent	Determined swelling in the subclavian fossa and on the arm	Not always	Not always
The state of deep reflexes	The inconsistent decline or revitalization on the arm, the absence of meningoradiculit is and tumors	Reduced in the shoulder area	Missing on hand	Reduced	Decrease due to swelling in the arm	Can be revitalized	Increased
Vascular and autonomic disorders	Absent or less pronounced with prolonged course of the disease	Absent	Cyanosis and brush strokes, brittle nails, thinning of	Swelling of the hand and area of edema is lower third of the forearm: smooth, shiny, cyanosis, cyanotic, cold.	The skin in the area of the brushes in the morning pastosity of	Moderate hyperhidrosis of the palms and feet,	Hyperemia of one half of the face, positive cold test,

		the skin	hyperemia, reduction of pulsation of the radial artery	Strengthening the venous pattern when lowering the hand				atrophy of the skin, nails, cardiac disturbances (sensation of "interruptions"),
Pain (trigger) zones	Interosseous, paravertebral in the affected area	In the area of the clavicle and shoulder	In the subclavian area		In the supraclavicular area		In the axillary region	Not typical	Sino-carotid zones in the region of cervical sympathetic ganglia
Sensitivity disorders	Unstable in the area of the affected root. Distinct in tumor	In the area of the shoulder, the forearm, chest and on elbow joint and hand	In the area of the forearm, the outside of the forearm, sometimes unsharp and hand	Hypesthesia in the form of a half-jacket	Unsharp paresthesias all over the arm, hypoesthesia in the hand area	Hypesesia in the wrist area in the morning	Hyposesthesia with hyperpathy in the form of a half-jacket as "burning hyperesthesia"

Differential diagnosis of lesions of the lumbosacral roots, plexus, lumbar spinal cord thickening and cauda equina

Type of injury	Etiological factors	Localization and nature of pain	Sensitivity disorders	Disorders of motor and reflexes	Vegetative and trophic disorders	Pelvic function status	X-ray changes	Changes in CSF	Blood changes
Lesion of lumbar roots: lumbar radiculopathy (sciatica)	Osteochondrosis (disc hernia). Injuries. Neurinoma rootlets and spine tumors (D12-L1). epidural abscess	Burning, sharp pain in the lumbar region radiating into the groin, thigh, knee joint, in the upper third of the external surface of the thigh, a positive symptom of Wasserman	Soreness of the paravertebral points of the lumbar region on the side of the lesion, radicular type of disorders. Possible hyperesthesia on the external surface of the lower leg and shin	The paresis of the muscles of the thigh, the raising of the leg and the extension of the leg are difficult. Decrease or extinction of the knee reflex	Hypotrophy or atrophy of hip muscles, acrocyanosis or dryness of the skin on the thigh	Not violated	Depends on the causes of compression. They can be typical for osteochondrosis, tumor, inflammatory changes in the D12-L1 region.	Protein-cell dissociation only with spinal cord tumors	Blood changes only with infection and compression
Lesion of lumbosacral	Osteochondrosis	Burning, sharp pain in	Hyperesthesia by the radicular type,	Limitation of	Protective one-sided	Not violated	Depends on the	Same	Same

The defeat of the lumbosacral roots: radiculopathy (radiculitis)	(hernia of the lumbosacral discs). Injuries. Anomalies of developement. Tumors of the spine, pelvic organs, in the paravertebral area, nadtechnik, epidural abscess	the lumbosacral portion with irradiation into the buttock, along the back surface of the leg. Pain is worse when the position changes, coughing, sneezing	tenderness of the paravertebral points and along the sciatic nerve. Positive tension symptom	movements and scoliosis in the lumbar region. Reduced strength in the muscles of the lower leg and foot. Revitalization of the knee reflex and extinction of the reflex from the heel	muscle tension in the lumbar region. Hypotrophy of the buttock muscles, tibia. Expressed hyperhidrosis on the leg, hair loss on the shin, the formation of trophic ulcers on the heel	ed cause of compression. The most common osteochondrosis, disc herniation, spondylolisthesis, developmental anomalies
The defeat of the gunshot	Injuries, gunshot	Injuries, gunshot	Tenderness at pressure on the	Flaccid paralysis or	Pain in the sacrum,	Not violated	Correspond to the	CSF changes same

21

lumbosacral plexus, lumbosacral plexitis	injuries, tumors coming from the pelvic organs and bones, diseases of the ovaries, vermiform appendage, psyt, epidural abscess	injuries, tumors coming from the pelvic organs and bones, diseases of the ovaries, vermiform	stomach, gluteal region and zones innervated by the femoral, sciatic and inhibitory nerves. Sensitivity disorders in zones innervated by the corresponding branches of the plexus	paresis of the muscles of the lower limb	atrophy of the leg muscle, buttocks, acrocyanosis, pastose, hair loss, hyperhidrosis, trophic ulcers on the sacrum and heel	only when the pathological process spreads to the spinal cord	nature of the spine and paravertebral structures of the near-vertebral organs and can be destructive, traumatic, tumor, infectious
The defeat of the coccygeal plexus (koktsigodiniya)	Traumas (microtrauma) of the sacrum, osteochondrosis, sacral tumors, sacroiliitis;	Burning, dull, persistent pain in the perineum and along the inner surface of the buttocks	Hypescension (anesthesia) or hyperesthesia in the perineum, anus, genitals, anesthesia of the inner surface of the hip,	With a combined lesion with the gluteal nerves, it is difficult to unbend the hip,	Not typical	In case of lesion of the osteochondrosis, consequences of coccyx injuries	Changes characteristic of lesion of genital and coccyx
						Without changes	Without changes

abscesses, pelvic organs diseases	the foot, which increases with prolonged sitting, with sexual intercourse	straighten the trunk when climbing the ladder. Weakness of the adductor muscles of the hip. the extinction of the cremaster and anal reflexes, the violation of the sexual function	geal plexuses, sacral region incontinence of urine and feces	of the sacral region and other diseases that cause coccicodinia

Differential and diagnostic signs of reflex vertebrogenic syndromes lumbosacral level

Name of the syndrome	Localization and pathogenesis	Complaints	Clinical manifestations	Diseases from which it is necessary to differentiate reflex syndromes	X-ray change	Necessary research
Lumbago	Pain in the lumbosacral region is due to strain or rupture of the fibrous ring	Sudden pain of the "lumbago" type, lasting for minutes, seconds or "tearing", pulsating, aggravated by coughing and sneezing	Antalgic position, fixed position of lumbar region, flatness of lordosis, kyphosis. The contraction of the muscles of the Livingstone triangle; reflex contracture of the square muscles of the back. Tendon reflexes are preserved, sensitivity is not	Can be self syndrome of osteochondrosis or the first (discalgic) stage of degenerative-dystrophic lesions - radicular syndrome	Spondylograms can be either only static changes, or signs of osteochondrosis, spondylosis. In some cases, the disk height may decrease	Spondylography in special projections after relief of pain syndrome

24

		upset			
Lumbalgia	Pain in the lumbar region occurs gradually with prolonged tension, cooling. The most common cause is neuro-osteo-fibrosis of interstitial ligaments, capsules of intervertebral joints, periarthrosis	Aching pain in the lower back, worse when the position of the body changes. Pain can spread to the buttock and to the leg	Static changes are less pronounced than with lumbago. Movement in the lumbar region is possible. Soreness in palpation of spinous processes, interstitial ligaments at the level of lesion. When you tilt back, the pain disappears, when you tilt forward - a sharp strain of the muscles of the back. Knee reflexes and reflexes from the calcaneal tendons	Osteoarthritis of the hip joint, sacroiliitis	Degenerative - dystrophic lesions of the spine. The symptom of the "strut" at the level of damage. The disk height can decrease	The same is the radiograph of the pelvis and the sacroiliac joint. General analysis of blood and urine. Myotonometry

25

Sciatica	Pain occurs due to irritation of fibrotic ring receptors and muscle connective tissue formations	Deep, squeezing pain in the buttock and hip joint, painful areas of radiating in the leg pain, increases with coughing, sneezing, change of position, chilliness or fever in the leg	When palpating trigger zones, neuro-osteo-fibrosis are noted; in muscles palpable rounded Cornelius nodules, densely elastic, without clear boundaries are preserved	Subacute stage of lumbosacral radiculitis, lumbago, lumbargia and sciatic nerve lesions	The same as with lumbago and lumbula
Pear-shaped muscle syndrome (pyriformis syndrome); the pear-shaped muscle sciatica	As a result of the compression of the neurovascular bundle between the pear-shaped muscle and the sacro-osteous ligament, sciatic nerve damage is formed. It is observed in osteochondrosis, spondyloarthrosis	Gradually there are pain in the gluteal region of the shin and foot, a feeling of paresthesias, chilliness; weakness in the leg when walking	Soreness in the palpation of the attachment points of the pear-shaped muscle to the medial surface of the large trochanter and to the lower part of the capsule of the sacroiliac joint. Bone's symptom	Inflammatory, tumoral, adhesive processes in the pelvis, leading to fibrosis or calcification of the pear-shaped mice. Radicular vertebrogenic syndrome, cocciogeny	Moderate manifestations of osteochondrosis, disorders of statics in the lumbosacral department	The same and reovasography of feet, thermometry, myotonometry	Radiography of the lumbosacral spine, pelvis cats. Examination of pelvic organs, rectum

MOTOR WEAKNESS

		is pain intensification with passive hip reduction over the middle line with simultaneous rotation of the inside.			
and secondary muscle damage in pathological processes in the pelvis					

Herniated discs of the lumbar spine
(mainly in men 30-50 years old, persons whose work is associated with constant flexion and extension of the spine

↓

Localization is most often LIV-LV, LIII-LIV

↓

CLINICAL PICTURE

Beginning: gradual build-up, initially dull, aching pain in the lumbar region, increasing with movement, muscle tension, lifting of heaviness, coughing, sneezing.

Course: the spread of pain to the buttock and the back or backside of the thigh or shin, on the side of the lesion (sciatica).

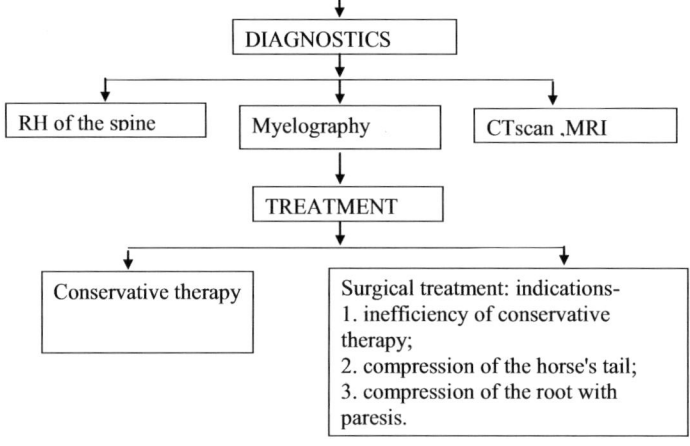

Backache
ANAMNESIS

1. localization of pain;
2. Irradiation of pain;
3. position of the body;
4. injury;
5. Indication of malignant neoplasms.

↓

GENERAL STUDY:

1. signs of infection;

2. signs of malignant neoplasm;
3. rectal examination (sphincter tone in the rectum).

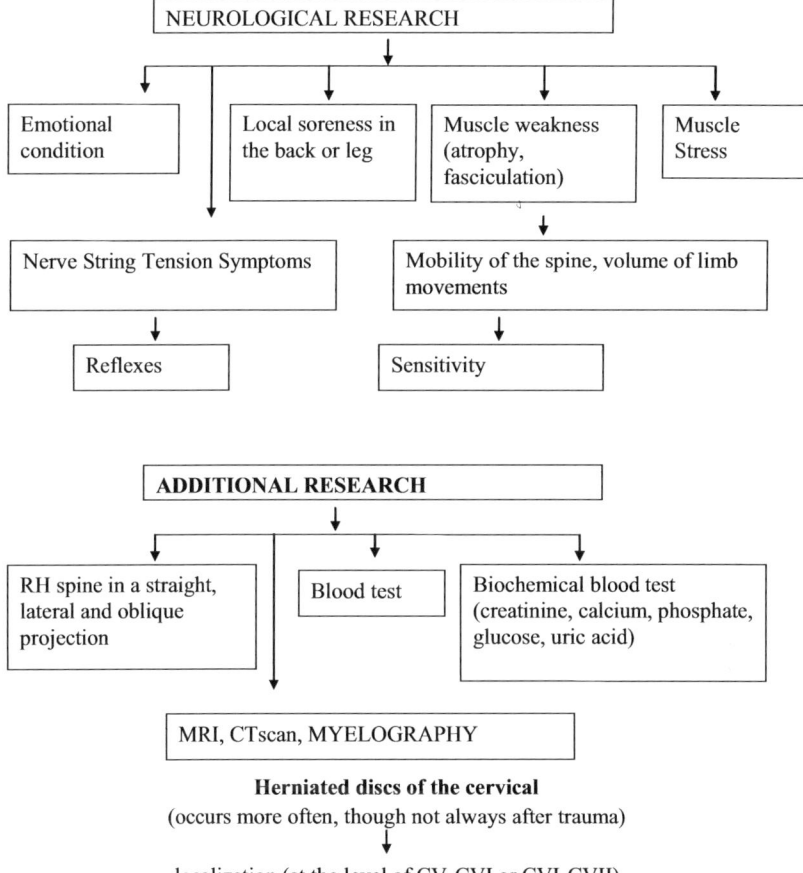

Herniated discs of the cervical
(occurs more often, though not always after trauma)

localization (at the level of CV-CVI or CVI-CVII)

Clinic: periodic pain in the posterior cervical region, tension of the paravertebral muscles, compression of the roots, irradiation of the pains, numbness and tingling in the innervation zone of the compressed root.

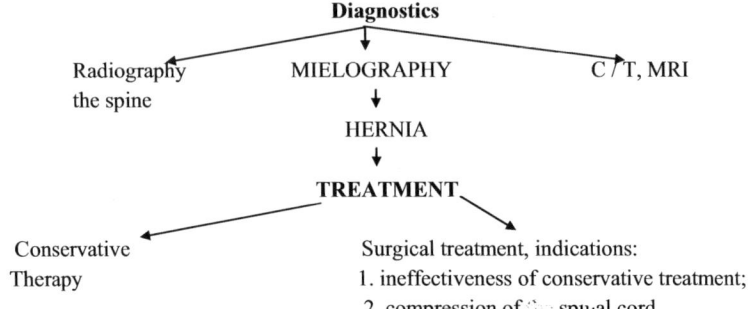

Schematic classification of vertebrogenic syndromes accompanied by pain

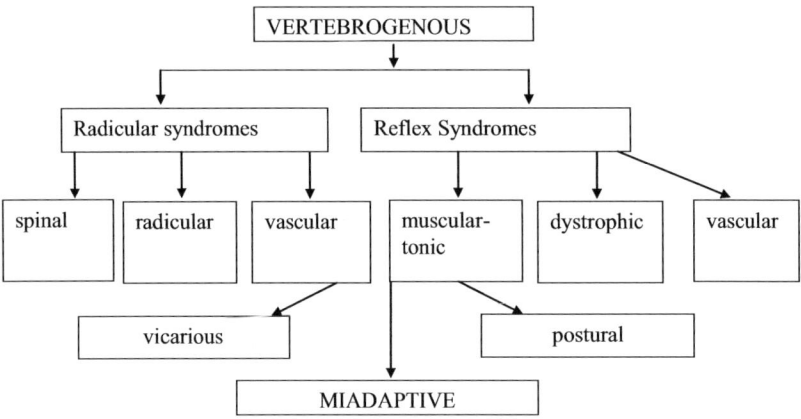

Features of patients' complaints, depending on the mechanism of stimulation of the sinuvertebral nerve receptors

Pain and factors affecting it	Mechanism of stimulation of the sinuvertebral nerve receptors in the affected PDS			
	Compress.	Dysfics.	The discourse	Inflammable.
The nature of pain	Acute	aching	aching	Breaking

Pain is aggravated	At the beginning of movement, coughing, sneezing	In the process of static loads, the longer the load, the more intense the pain	In the rest position	During sleep, because of pain, it wakes up
Pain is aggravated	At rest, sometimes in a certain position	When the load terminates	When driving	When moving, kneading, rubbing the affected area
Other Features			The pain is accompanied by a burning sensation, chilliness in the affected spine	During the day, the pain decreases and sometimes the patient feels almost healthy in the evening

Information on objective characteristics, characteristic for various mechanisms of stimulation of the sinuvertebral nerve receptors in the sporadic vertebral segment (VS)

Symptoms	The mechanism of stimulation of the sinuvertebral nerve receptors in the affected vertebral-motor segment (VS)			
	Compress.	Dysfics.	The discourse	Inflammable.
Vertebral Deformation	Expressed or expressed sharply, most often in the form of kyphoscoliotic or hyperlordoscoliotic	Pronounced insignificantly, usually in the sagittal plane (kyphosis or hyperlordosis)	Slightly expressed	Expressed in the morning, in the evening less
Myofixation	Sharply expressed	Slightly expressed at the onset of an exacerbation and abruptly at the end	Slightly expressed	Pronounced in the morning and mildly expressed in the evening

Pain during palpation	Most expressed in one point of the affected VDS	Uniform of all ligament-articular structures of the affected VS	Uniform of all ligament-articular structures of the affected VS	Several VS s in the joint area
Symptoms of extension and flexion in the affected vertebral column	Strongly expressed	Expressed	Slightly expressed	Pronounced in the morning, in the evening slightly expressed
Surface sensitivity in the area of the affected vertebral column	Not changed	Not changed	Hypesesia	Hypesesia

Information on the symptoms characteristic of various extrovertebral syndromes

	Extravertebral syndromes			
	Muscular		Neural	Neurovascular
	Dystonic	Dystrophic		
The nature of pain	pulling	lustrous	lustrous	lustrous
Paresthesia	no	In the dermato-me	In the dermato-me	In the zone of vascularization of the wounded vessel
Factors that increase complaints	Motor loads			Change in ambient temperature

Objective symptoms Inspection	Objective symptoms Inspection		Atrophy and hypotrophy can occur in the myotome	Change in the coloration of skin integuments, shades may be local
The volume of movements in the affected limb	Changed	Changed	Changed	Not changed
Muscle tone	Enhanced	Raised or lowered	Raised or lowered	Not changed
Consistency of muscles	Local hypertonia	Local hypertonia	Hypotrophy	Not changed
Vascular tone	Not changed	Not changed	Not changed	Changed
Sensitivity change	Not changed	In the affected quadrant	In dermatome or sclerotome	Sometimes in the distal zones of the limb

Symptoms typical for various complications of biomechanical sanogenetic reactions

Symptoms	Complications				
	Primary			Secondary	
	Muscular	Ligamentous-articular	Bony	The neural	Vessels
Complaints	Aching, aching, pulling pains outside the primary lesion zone, intensifying with loads on the affected vertebral column	Shooting intermittent Deep or permanent permanent pain in distal areas	Periodic or persistent pain in and out of the vertebrae, exacerbated by stress	To pains of a different nature in the zone of localization of primary complications, numbness, stasis, weakness in the zone of the limbs	
Objectively	Morbidity of the non-	Soreness in ligaments and	Painfulness of bone	The change in muscle	Change in vascular

Palpation	rhythmic muscle in muscles	joints	formations	tone, in the innervation of which a paroxysmal nerve or plexus takes part	tone
Sensitivity	Changed by quadrant type			Changed in the zone of innervation of the affected nerve or plexus	It can be changed in the distal form of the coordinates
Inspection	-	-	Swelling in the area of the affected bone		Swelling in the area of the affected bone

Treatment of osteochondrosis of the lumbar spine.
Koreshkovo-compression syndrome.

Acute period	Subacute Period	Chronic period
Painkillers NSAIAs - ksefokam in a dose of 8 mg 1-2 times a day. in / in, / m, as the pain subsides - peros 4-8 mg 2 times a day for 7 days, diclofenac 2 ml in / m. Muscular relaxants-sirdalud 4 mg or myolastane 50 mg. Antidepressants. Dehydrating agents. Novocaine (paravertebral) blockades. Dimexide	NSAIAs (xifokam diclofenac, nimesulide, voltaren), Vascular Physiotherapy Locomasi, gels, dimexid applications	Vitamins gr. HF. Exercise therapy Massage Acupuncture Physiotherapy

applications are topical, ointments, gels. Physiotherapy		

Treatment of osteochondrosis of the cervical spine

Acute period	Subacute Period	Chronic period
Painkillers NSAIAs - ksefokam 8 mg * 1-2 times per day. in / in, / m, as the pain subsides peros 4-8 mg * 2 times a day for 7 days, diclofenac Muscular relaxants-sirdalud (2-4mg.) Dehydrating Local applications of dimexide, ointments, gels Physiotherapy Antidepressants, with vertebral artery syndrome vasoactive drugs, betagistins	NSAIAs (xefokam, diclofenac, voltaren) Local applications of dimexide, ointments, gels Physiotherapy With dizziness betagistiny, vasoactive drugs	Group B vitamins, exercise therapy Massage Acupuncture Physiotherapy

Neuralgia of the trigeminal nerve - Phosergil's disease, NEVRALGIA QVINTI MAJOR

Classification:
I. Primary
II. Symptomatic.

I. Primary (esentional) neuralgia of the trigeminal nerve.

Sick people older (after 40 years) and more often women.

In the clinical picture of trigeminal neuralgia, there are usually 5 main features.

1. Severe localization of pain in the territory innervated by the trigeminal nerve to the right or left, or in the innervation zone of one of the branches of the trigeminal nerve. Most often in zone II of the branch (suborbital nerve), less often in the third branch (the chin nerve) and even more rarely in the I branch (supraorbital nerve). Each attack begins with the same territory and only later can spread to the territory of other, neighboring branches of the trigeminal nerve.

2. Paroxysmal flow and the nature of pain. The pains of a drilling, pulling character are most often in the skin, in the mucosa or both, less often in the teeth for several seconds to several tens of seconds, followed by a period of extinction of the pain attack, which in turn is prolonged up to several tens of seconds. The total duration of the attack is up to 1.5-2 minutes. During the attack, the patient freezes in a painful grimace, the facial muscles of the face are more often in a state of tonic contraction, may be hypersalivation, increased lacrimation, Nazarene.

3. The provoked nature of seizures with the presence of trigger trigger zone, the zone of the trigger, the irritation of which (conversation, mimicry, palpation, eating, shaving, even a simple smile) can cause an attack. Most often, the skin is in the area of the nasolabial fold, upper lip, wings of the nose, less often the eyebrow and other areas. It should be noted that a strong irritation of this zone (strong pressure or prick in the study of sensitivity) does not cause an attack and is transferred safely.

4. Immediately after the attack, there is a refractory period lasting up to several minutes, when the presence of irritation of the cortical zone does not cause a new attack and which patients are used in severe cases to take food or produce a toilet face.

5. Lack of objective data for neurological examination during the inter-attack period.

II. Symptomatic

Trigeminal pains or symptomatic trigeminal neuralgia of the V nerve (Raeder's syndrome, Kosten's syndrome, with syringobulbia, in organic processes in the cerebellar angle: tumors, inflammatory processes, vascular aneurysms, etc.).

Clinical picture.

The closest sign of symptomatic neuralgia that causes it to differentiate from the true trigeminal neuralgia is the trigeminal localization of pain, which can correspond to the topography of the innervation of the trigeminal nerve.

However, the other three classic features: the paroxysmal character provoking the character of pain with the presence of trigger zones, the absence of objective data for a neurological examination - no, or they do not have those features that are characteristic of true neuralgia.

Pain more often constant, less intensive, start zones are not defined. There are objective symptoms: a decrease in the corneal reflex, hypoesthesia, the pathology of the motor portion of the trigeminal nerve, or other craniocerebral (VI, VII, VIII, IX, X, XI, XII).

Treatment of trigeminal neuralgia

I. Drug therapy.

The most effective finlepsin (carbamazepine) - an average dose of 600-800 mg, maintaining a dose of 200 mg. A positive effect is observed in 80% of patients (60% - withdrawal of seizures and 20% - improvement).

Less effective piknoleptsin (suksilen) - 0.25 to 4 times and maintenance dose 1 time per day; trimetin - 0.2 g 3-4 times a day, maintenance dose 1 time per day.

II. Acupuncture.

III. Also blockades with novocaine of separate branches of the trigeminal nerve in the channels of exit to the face with a therapeutic and diagnostic purpose are also applied.

IV. Alcoholization of the same branches of the trigeminal nerve with 70% alcohol (alcoholization of the gasserous node), directed hydrothermal destruction of the sensitive trigeminalroot (author L.Ya. Livshits).

Surgery.
- Neurotomy of the spine of the trigeminal nerve in the bridge of the cerebellum above the gasserous node.
- Stereotoxic destruction of the descending spine of the trigeminal nerve in the medulla oblongata.
- Microvascular decompression of the trigeminal nerve root.
- Percutaneous radiofrequency destruction of the trigeminal nerve roots.
- In recent years, new approaches have appeared in the treatment of trigeminal neuralgia:
- Stereotactic radiosurgery (gamma-knife) is a bloodless method of destroying the sensitive spine with the help of focused gamma radiation.
- Epidural neurostimulation of the motor cortex of the brain

Neuropathy of the facial nerve

MAIN SYMPTOMS:

Prozoparesis, prozoplegia, lagophthalmus, positive Bell symptom, a symptom of "eyelashes", a decrease in the superciliary and corneal reflex.

CLINICAL PICTURE, depending on the level of affection of the VII pair:

priporazheniiya-prozoplegia napinegopravleniya, defeat VIparyyvodniknikovyh way of the bridge (alternatingmodernyMyyara-Guberai of Fovil)

when the spine is injured in the bridge of the bridge, prozoplegia, hearing loss, impaired taste on the front 2/3 of the tongue and dry eyes

with lesion of the nerve trunk in the facial canal (before the departure of the large stony nerve), - prozoplegia, dry eyes, hyperacusia, a disorder of taste and salivation

with a lesion of the nerve below the retraction of the stenal nerve and above the tympanic-prozoplegia string, lacrimation, taste and salivation disorders

when the nerve is damaged below the retraction of the tympanic string or after exiting the stylophyllar opening, prozoplegia, lachrymation.

Syndrome of facial nerve damage at various levels

Level of defeat	Paralysis of the muscles of the face	Reduction of brow and corneal reflexes	Lachrymatince on	Disturbance of taste on the front 2/3 of the tongue	Reduction of salivation	Hyperacusis	Dry eyes	Hearing loss	Vestibular disorders
In the region of the stylophyllum orifice	+	+	-	-	-	-	-	-	-
In the front channel is higher than the retraction of the drum string	+	+	+	+	+	-	-	-	-
In the facial canal above the stent nerve	+	+	+	+	+	+	-	-	-
In the facial canal above the stent nerve	+	+	-	+	+	+	+	-	-
In the facial canal above the stent nerve	+	+	-	+	+	-	+	+	+

39

Treatment of facial nerve neuropathy

In an acute period, glucocorticoid therapy with anti-edematous, antihistamine and immunosuppressive properties is indicated. In the first three days of the acute period, in the absence of contraindications, hydrocortisone is injected intravenously into 125 hydrocortisone at a dose of 125 units 2 times a day, then prednisolone is administered internally, starting from 40 mg / day with progressive decreasing doses, the course of treatment lasts 2 -3 weeks.

Penicillin, 24 million units / day, is prescribed for otogennogo lesions facial. Antiviral agents are prescribed for the treatment of herpetic etiology. Dehydration agents, vasodilators (1% of nicotinic acid 1.0, theonikol, etc.). Frequently, vitamins of group B.Violation-UFO or electric field of UHF are widely used in the stage of the disease. From 4-5 days of the disease, phonophoresis of hydrocortisone or ultrasound is prescribed. On the area of the exit of the facial nerve application of dimexide, which is able to penetrate deeply into the tissues and give a protivoprotechny, anti-inflammatory and vasodilating effect.

After 7-10 days from the onset of the disease, massage, exercise therapy, electrophoresis of medicines are added: 0.1% of prozerin, nivalin, or 0.05% of dibazol.

After a lapse of a month from the beginning of the disease, mud, paraffin or ozocerite applications are prescribed.

Significant application of prenieuropathies of the facial nerve was found by acupuncture.

When the first signs of post-paralytic contracture appear, it is necessary to cancel the electro-therapy with anticholinesterase drugs. It is prescribed carbamazepine (finlepsin) in a dose-free 100-600 mg / day. Application mud is recommended on the collar zone.

POLYNEUROPATHY

Risk factors for polyneuropathy:
- Chronic intoxication (use of alcohol, drugs, drugs, poisoning with arsenic, lead);
- endocrine diseases (diabetes mellitus);
- metabolic factors (hypo- and avitaminosis B1, B12, renal pathology);
- malignant neoplasms;
- autoimmune diseases (rheumatoid arthritis, SLE, SVD, and other.);
- varicose veins, and other

Classification of polyneuropathies (Levin O.S, 2006)
According to the etiology
1. Idiopathic inflammatory / non-inflammatory polyneuropathies-Guillain-Barre syndrome, chronic inflammatory demyelinating polyradiculoneuropathy (CIDP), chronic idiopathic axonal polyneuropathy

2. Polyneuropathies with metabolic disorders and eating disorders - diabetic polyneuropathy, polyneuropathies with other endocrine diseases, uremic polyneuropathy, hepatic polyneuropathy, polyneuropathies with a deficiency of vitamins

3. Polyneuropathies with exogenous intoxications - alcoholic polyneuropathy, polyneuropathies with intoxication by other substances, medicinal polinzvropatii

4. Polyneuropatii with systemic diseases - dysproteinemic polyneuropathies, polyneuropathy with sarcoidosis, polyneuropathy in diffuse connective tissue diseases and vasculitis

5. Polyneuropathies in infectious diseases and vaccinations - infectious-toxic half-neuropathies (with diphtheria), postinfectious polyneuropathies (in case of epidemic parotitis, measles, infectious mononucleosis, influenza, VID infection, neuroborreliosis)

6. Polyneuropathies with malignant neoplasms

7. Hereditary polyneuropathies

By pathogenesis
There are three main types of polyneuropathy:
1. caused by primary axon lesions (axonal polyneuropathies)
2. caused by the primary lesion of the myelin sheaths (demyelinating polyneuropathies),
3. caused by primary damage to cells of peripheral neurons (neuronopathy)

CLINIC
According to prevailing clinical signs
1. Motor (motor),
2. Sensitive (sensory),
3. The vegetative,
4. Mixed

By the nature of the distribution of the lesion
1. Distal (symmetrical) involvement of all limbs;
2. Involvement of all parts of the upper and / or lower limbs;

3. Multiple neuropathies with predominantly proximal lesions;
4. Involvement of cranial nerves

Clinical manifestations of polyneuropathic syndrome
1. Pain
2. Paresthesia
3. Muscle weakness
4. Hypotrophy, hypotension
5. Decreased reflexes
6. Sensitivity disorders by the type of "gloves or sock"

Syndromology of polyneuropathies is determined by signs of defeat:

1. The motor system - weakness and atrophy of the muscles of the extremities and torso.
2. The reflex sphere is the animation, and then the extinction of the tendon, periosteal and skin reflexes.
3. Sensitive system - hyperpathy and dysesthesia, followed by a decrease and loss of surface and deep sensitivity in the distal parts of the extremities, according to the polyneuric type.
4. Vegetative disorders - local circulatory disorders and lymphatic flow, thermoregulation, sweating, trophic disorders.

The main clinical manifestations of polyneuropathies (Levin O.S, 2006)

symptoms	negative	positive
motor	muscle weakness (usually tetraparesis or lower paraparesis) muscle hypotension muscle atrophy, areflexia	tremor crump fascicle neuro myotonia
sensory	hypesthesia, paresthesia sensitive ataxia	Hyperesthesiology syndrome restless legs
vegetative	orthostatic hypotension fixed pulse weakening of motor function gastrointestinal tract hyperreflexia of urinary bladder	arterial hypertension tachycardia intestinal colic Irritated bladder hyperhidrosis

	hypohidrosyl anhidrosis impotence	

Clinically, demyelinating polyneuropathies are characterized by:
- early prolapse of tendon reflexes;
- pronounced violation of joint-muscular and vibration sensitivity and, accordingly, pronounced sensitive ataxia with relative safety of pain and *temperature sensitivity;*
- involvement of both distal and proximal limb sections (demyelinating polyneuropathies often affect proximal segments of nerve fibers, including spinal roots);
- more pronounced and common paresis, but less gross atrophy of the muscles.

Comparative characteristics of axonal and demyelinating polyneuropathies (Levin O.S, 2006)

symptoms	axonal polyneuropathies	demyelinating polyneuropathies
Start	gradual, subacute, less often acute	acute, subacute or gradual
distribution of symptoms	predominantly distal parts of the extremities	Both distal and proximal parts of the extremities are involved
tendon reflexes	may remain intact (especially in the proximal part)	early fall or fall out
amyotrophy	early	develops later
disturbance of pain and temperature sensitivity	can be expressed	usually mild or moderate
depressive disorder	rare	can be expressed
autonomic dysfunction	expressed	moderate
recovery rate	for months or years	within 6 to 10 weeks
incomplete recovery	often	often
cerebrospinal fluid	protein level within normal limits	often protein-cell dissociation
data of EMG	signs of demyelination:	signs of demyelination:

	decrease in the rate of "increasing distal latency, changing 1-response, blocks of conduct and dispersion Denervation signs appear relatively late	decrease in the rate of "increasing distal latency, changing 1-response, blocks of conduct and dispersion Denervation signs appear relatively late

Polyneuropathies with damage to sensory fibers of different caliber (LevinO.S, 2006)

	Polyneuropathies with predominant lesion of thick sensory fibers	Polyneuropathies with predominant involvement of thin sensory fibers
main manifestations	complaints of numbness, paresthesia, a feeling of "vatnosti", a violation of deep sensitivity, early loss of succinic reflexes, a sensitive ataxia	complaints of burning pain, disturbances of pain and temperature sensitivity with hyperesthesia and allodynia, tendon reflexes can be preserved, autonomic dysfunction
diseases	diabetic poly-neuropathy, diphtheria poly-neuropathy, acute sensory (atactic) poly-neuropathy, CVDP (sensory form) disproteinemic polyneuropathy, polyneuropathy with biliary cirrhosis	diabetic polyneuropathy, alcoholic polyneuropathy, amyloid polyneuropathy, Polyneuropathy associated with VID infection, polyneuropathy in sarcoidosis, hereditary sensory-vegetative neuropathies, Fabry's disease

Polyneuropathies with severe pain syndrome (Levin O.S, 2006)
Idiopathic (cryptogenic) polyneuropathies
Diabetic polyneuropathy.
Alcoholic polyneuropathy
Amyloid polyneuropathy

Guillain-Barre Syndrome
Paraneoplastic polyneuropathy
Polyneuropathy in sarcoidosis
Uremic polyneuropathy
Medicinal polyneuropathies (caused by metronidazole,
nitrofurans, suramin, taxol, thalidomide, nucleosides)
Toxic polyneuropathies (caused by arsenic, thallium)
Alimentary polyneuropathies (with a deficiency of vitamins B1 B6, B12,
pantothenic acid)
Polyneuropathy associated with VID infection
Polyneuropathy (meningoradiculoneuropathy) with tick-borne borreliosis
Leprosy
Polyneuropathy (multiple mononeuropathy) in vasculitis
Porphyria polyneuropathy
Hereditary sensory-vegetative neuropathies
Fabry's disease
Tangier disease

Polyneuropathies with pronounced vegetative manifestations

Idiopathic polyneuropathies
Acute dysimmune vegetative neuropathies
Acute pandisavanomia
Acute cholinergic autonomic neuropathy
Vegetative neuropathy with Guillain-Barre syndrome
Chronic idiopathic autonomic neuropathy
Cholinergic (associated with antibodies to choline receptors
vegetative ganglia) Adrenergic
Chronic idiopathic anhidrosis
Metabolic polyneuropathies
Diabetic polyneuropathy
Polyneuropathy in primary systemic amyloidosis
Uremic polyneuropathy
Hepatic polyneuropathy
Polyneuropathy in chronic lung diseases
Thiamine-deficient polyneuropathy
Toxic polyneuropathies

Alcoholic polyneuropathy
Polyneuropathy with medicinal intoxications (vincristine, cisplatin, amiodarone)
Polyneuropathy when poisoned with metals (thallium, arsenic, mercury)
Polyneuropathies with poisoning with organic solutions
Polyneuropathy in case of poisoning with other toxic substances (acrylamide, and other.)
Infectious polyneuropathies
Diphtheria polyneuropathy
Polyneuropathies associated with VID infection
Leprosy
Polyneuropathy in tick-borne borreliosis
Polyneuropathies in malignant neoplasms
Paraneoplastic disautonomy
Enteric neuropathy (pseudo-ileus)
Vegetative neuropathy with Lambert-Ito-n syndrome
Polyneuropathies in systemic diseases
Polyneuropathies in diffuse diseases of connective tissue (rheumatoid arthritis, SLE, Sjogren's syndrome, systemic scleroderma)
Polyneuropathy with inflammatory bowel disease (disease Crohn's disease, ulcerative colitis)
Hereditary polyneuropathies.
Porphyria
Family amyloid neuropathy Hereditary sensory-vegetative neuropathy Neuropathy associated with a deficiency of dopamine-beta-hydroxylase
Fabry's disease

Involvement of cranial nerves in polyneuropathies of various etiologies (Y. Harati, 1995, with changes)

diseases	often involved cranial nerves	more rarely involved cranial nerves
Guillain-Barre Syndrome	VI, VII	
Miller Fischer Syndrome	III, IV, VI	
Diabetes	III	IV, VI, VII
Diphtheria	IX	II, III

Sarcoidosis	VII	I, III, IV, V, VI
CKB	V	
Porphyria	VII, X	III, IV, V, XI, XII
Disease of Refsum	I, VIII	
Amyloidosis	V	
Arsenic poisoning	V	

Additional methods of investigation in patients with polyneuropathy (Levin O.S, 2006)

method of investigation	excluded diseases
clinical blood test	Inflammatory diseases diffuse connective tissue diseases blood diseases malignant neoplasm lead poisoning
study of blood sugar level test for glucose tolerance	diabetes impaired glucose tolerance
a study of the level of urea and creatinine in the blood	kidney disease
hepatic tests	liver disease alcoholism
a study of the level of thyroid hormones and TSH in the blood	hypothyroidism
Serum electrophoresis of serum / urine immunoelectrophoresis	paraproteinemia diffuse connective tissue diseases
rheumatological tests (rheumatoid factor, antinuclear antibodies, circulating immune complexes and other.)	diffuse connective tissue diseases systemic vasculitis
a study of the level of vitamin B | 2, folic acid, thiamine in the blood	vitamin deficiency
serological tests	postinfectious polyneuropathies
toxicological screening (gas chromatography, and other.)	intoxication
study of urinary excretion of porphobilinogen and aminolevulinic acid	porphyria
Radiography (chest, abdominal organs, spine, pelvis, skull, and other.)	malignant neoplasms osteolytic and osteosclerotic myeloma

ultrasound examination of the abdominal cavity endoscopic examination of the gastrointestinal tract	malignant neoplasms
radioisotope scintigraphy	myeloma, bone metastases
bone marrow biopsy	leukemia, myeloma, macroglobulinemia, Waldenstrom

During the polyneuropathy, regardless of the etiological factors that caused it, and pathogenetic processes that cause the development of symptoms, we can distinguish several stages:
1. Latent period
2. Acute period-1-1.5 months from the onset of the disease
3. Early recovery period - up to 2-3 months from the start diseases
4. Recovery period-up to 1 year from the onset of the disease
5. The period of residual phenomena

General directions of therapy

I. Immunocorrective therapy

II. Detoxification therapy
Transfusion of detoxification drugs: reamberin, and other.
1. Treatment with complexones: unitiol, kurenyl, sodium thiosulfate.
2. Extracorporeal detoxification: hemosorption, hemodialysis.
3. Enterosorption: reception of sorbents.

III. Antihypoxiant and vascular therapy
1. Hyperbaric oxygenation (HBO).
2. Indirect antihypoxants: alpha-tocopherol, ascorbic acid,
3. Glutamic acid, alpha-lipoic acid (thiogamma).
4. Drugs that improve microcirculation: rheopolyglucin, pentoxifylline, cavinton, nicergoline, compliance.
5. Angioprotectors: venorurton, anginin, dicinone, doxium, ascorbic acid, rutin, calcium preparations.

IV. Neurometabolic therapy
1. Nootropic drugs: piracetam, instenon, encephabol, pantogam.
2. Neuroprotective: vitamins of group B

3. Metabolic drugs: riboksin, cytochrome C, actovegin, cerebrolysin, lipostabil, and other.
4. Anabolic steroids.
5. Non-steroidal anabolics.
V. Rehabilitation therapy
1. Anticholinesterase drugs.
2. Physiotherapeutic, balneological procedures and exercise therapy.
3. Hyperbaric oxygenation.
VI. Symptomatic therapy

Infectious diseases of the nervous system
Diagnostic algorithm of meningeal syndrome

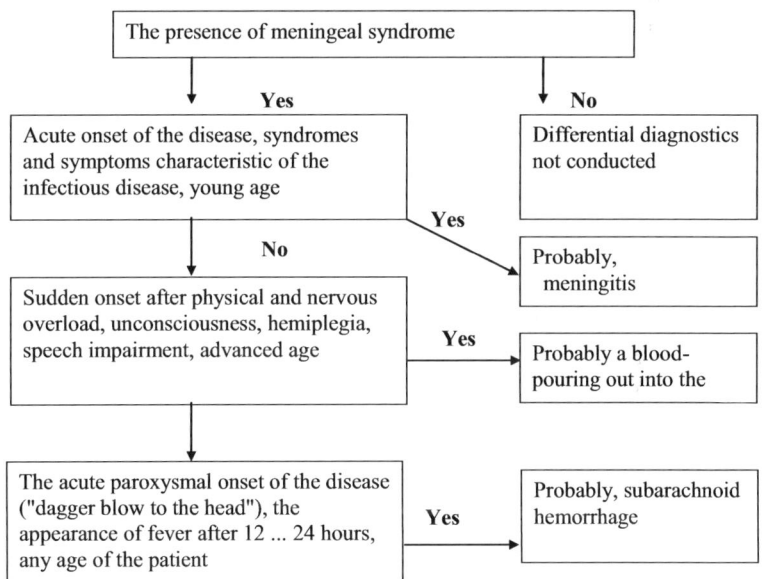

Algorithm of diagnostic search in the presence of a patient with meningeal and cerebral symptoms

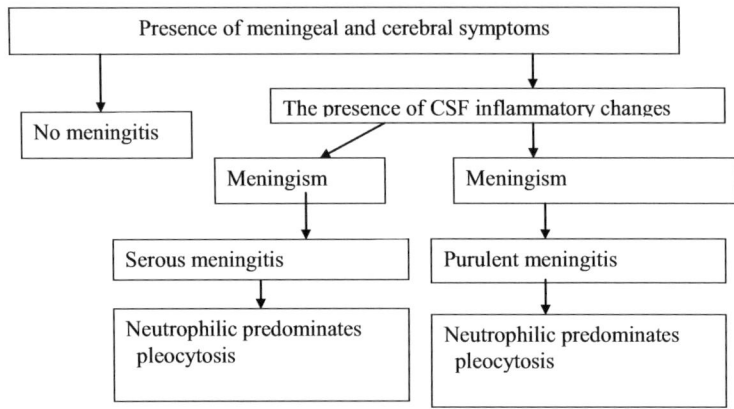

Scheme of classification of serous meningitis (infectious)

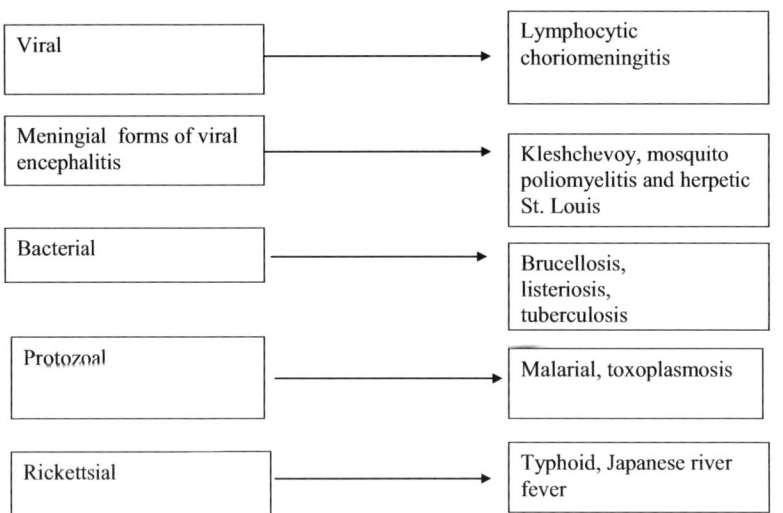

| Spirochelous | → | Syphilitic, leptospiral |

| Fungal | | Blastomycosis |

→

| Helminth | | Ascaridosis |

Scheme of classification of serous meningitis (non-infectious)

| With traumatic brain injury | ↔ | With direct exposure through cerebral pathways |

| With tumors of the brain | ↔ | With lead and arsenico-viscous intoxication |

| With subarachnoid hemorrhage | ↔ | When endolumbular administration of drugs |

| When contrasting the cerebrospinal fluid |

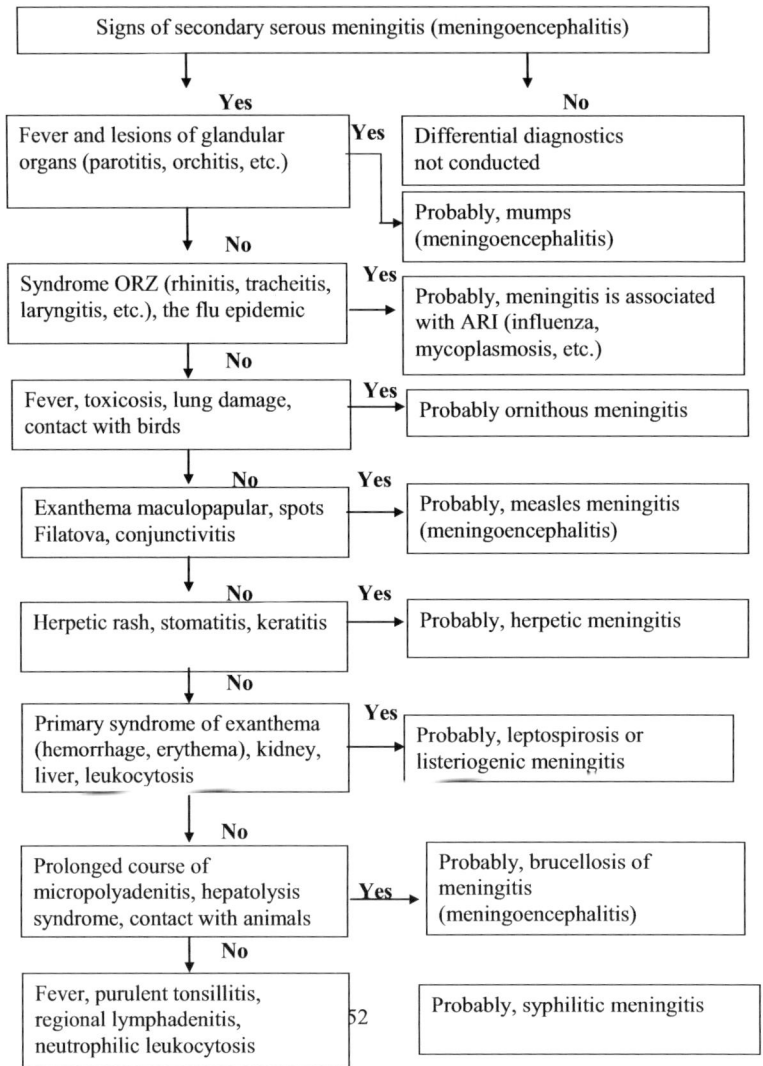

Yes →

Algorithm of diagnostic search in the presence of a patient signs of meningitis

```
┌─────────────────────────────────────────────┐
│   The presence of clinical signs of meningism │
└─────────────────────────────────────────────┘
```

Condition		Probable diagnosis
Fever and ARD syndrome (rhinitis, pharyngitis, tracheitis)	Yes →	Differential diagnostics not conducted. Probably, meningococcal nasopharyngitis with meningism
↓		
Acute onset, fever, expressed nasopharyngitis, leukocytosis	Yes →	Probably infectious mononucleosis with meningism
↓		
Fever, tonsillitis, lymphadenopathy, hepatolienal syndrome, mononuclear leukocytosis	→	Probably, angina with meningism
↓ No		
Fever, purulent tonsillitis, regional lymphadenitis, neutrophilic leukocytosis	Yes →	Probably, salmonellosis with meningism
↓		
Fever sharp gastroenteritis	Yes →	Probably acute dysentery with meningism
↓		
A delayed onset, fever, hemocolitis	Yes →	Probably, leptospirosis or listeriosis meningitis
↓ No		
A gradual onset, a fever, a roseolous rash from the 7th ... 9th day, hepatolienal syndrome	Yes →	Probably, typhoid fever with meningism

Early (in the first 2 days) diagnosis of meningococcal meningitis and tactics of hospitalization of patients

The most diagnostic signs

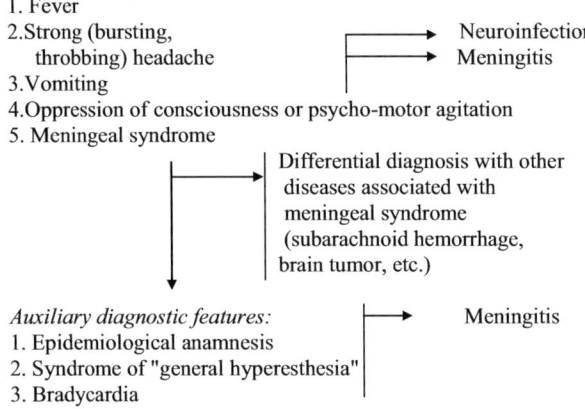

1. Fever
2. Strong (bursting, throbbing) headache → Neuroinfection? Meningitis
3. Vomiting
4. Oppression of consciousness or psycho-motor agitation
5. Meningeal syndrome
   → Differential diagnosis with other diseases associated with meningeal syndrome (subarachnoid hemorrhage, brain tumor, etc.)

Auxiliary diagnostic features:
1. Epidemiological anamnesis → Meningitis
2. Syndrome of "general hyperesthesia"
3. Bradycardia

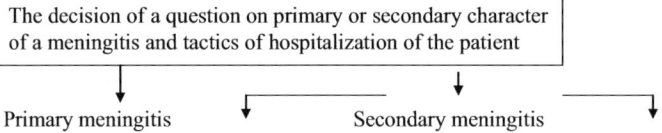

The decision of a question on primary or secondary character of a meningitis and tactics of hospitalization of the patient

Primary meningitis   Secondary meningitis

Decisive diagnostic signs:
1 Results of the study of cerebrospinal fluid.
2 Bacteriological study of cerebrospinal fluid, blood, nasopharyngeal mucus.

Meningococcal meningitis (cerebro-spinal epidemic meningitis)

1. Epidemiological features	-winter-spring period (February-April)
	¬ significant contagiosity
	-Conclusion during periods of outbreaks of acute

	respiratory disease -the contact with a patient with meningococcal nasopharyngitis, meningitis, a healthy meningococcus predominantly children
2. Transmission path	-air-drip
3. Incubation period	1-5 days
4. Development	-shaped
5. Body temperature	39-40
6. Prevailing symptoms	meningeal symptoms
7. Headache	Sharp, strongest
8. Vomiting	frequent multiple

Urgent hospitalization in an infectious hospital	Meningitis as a manifestation of another infectious disease (leptospirosis, mumps). Pneumococcal meningitis	Meningitis as a complication in diseases: ENT organs, surgical, urological, tuberculosis, syphilis	Urgent hospitalization in the corresponding "etiology" of the disease-noninfectious hospital

9. Meningeal symptoms	develop by the end of 1-day, MAX on the 2nd day
10. Encephalitic symptoms	expressed meningoencephalitis in 10% of patients, pyramidal signs, the severity of III, V, more-VI, VII pairs of CN

Meningococcal meningitis

11. Changes found outside the nervous system	on 2-3days herpes labialis, herpes nazalis, herpes lingualis- Pathognomonic hemorrhagic petechial and purple rash.chasche on the trunk and lower limbs (buttocks, hips, shins)

12. Early complication	acute cerebral edema secondary trunk syndrome - acute adrenal insufficiency (Waterhouse-Friderixen syndrome
13. Likvor	- turbid, sharply positive protein assays, high neutrophilic pleyocytosis, increased pressure -tank. study-meningococcus Vekselbauma -Sitting from CSF-the same
14. Blood	non-trophic leukocytosis with a leftward shift, an increase in ESR
15. Consequences	hydrocephalus -Dement -amaurosis
16. Duration of the disease	- hydrocephalus -Dement -amaurosis
17. Outcome	recovery in 90-95% of cases

Staphylococcal and streptococcal meningitis

1. Epidemiological features	complication of extracranial purulent process
2. Transmission path	is often a consequence of sepsis
3. Development	-Hematogenic
4. Body temperature	-contact
5. Headache	- sudden, rapid
6. Encephalitic symptoms	-40
7. Changes found outside the nervous system	-Intense
8. Early complication	From the beginning of the disease, delirium, depression of consciousness, down to coma. Severe focal symptomatology, convulsions.
9. Liquor	-Symptoms of sepsis: lowering blood pressure, enlarging the liver and spleen, deafness of the heart tones.

Meningitis caused by Pseudomonas aeruginosa

1. Epidemiological features	-expressing sepsis or superinfection in children and adults after surgery
2. Primary symptoms	-heavy meningoencephalitis with a tendency to the formation of pioencephalitis
3. Likvor	-green-bluish color, increased protein, reduced sugar, high neutrophilic cytosis -Association-Pseudomonas aeruginosa
4. Techenie	-shot with a quick fatal outcome -more long undulating
5. Transmission Path	-Hematogenic

Pneumococcal meningitis

1. Epidemiological features	- Complication of diseases caused by pneumococcus (pneumonia, purulent otitis, tracheobronchitis)
2. Transmission Path	-Hematogenic
3. Development	-shaped
4. Body temperature	up to 40 and above
5. Primary symptoms	pronounced meningeal symptoms
6. Headache	The sharpest
7. Vomiting	Multiple
8. Meningeal symptoms	develop at the end of 1-2 days.
9. Encephalitic symptoms	often meningoencephalitis: clonic-tonic convulsions, various forms of impaired consciousness, paralysis of limbs, ataxia, hyperkinesia, lesion III, less often - VII, IX, X pairs of CN
10. Changes that are found outside the nervous system	Hemorrhagic rash

11. Likvor	cloudy greenish-gray, high neutrophilic pleocytosis, a slight increase in pressure, an increase in the protein to 3-6 g / l and>, neutrophilic cytosis from 0.01-10 / 9 l, fibrinoid precipitate, a decrease in sugar
12. Blood	-About investigation-pneumococcus
13. Duration of the disease	-Sitting from CSF-the same
14. Expenditure	recovery in the treatment of underlying disease

Purulent meningitis caused by Afanasyev's haemophilic rod (influenza-meningitis)

1. Epidemiological features	- especially children from 6 months are ill. up to 4 years Complications of bronchitis, pneumonia, otitis
2. Transmission Path	-Hematogenic
3. The period of incubation	Fast
4. Development	-astropic, 20-25% of the time
5. Body temperature	37-40
6. Primary symptoms	general infectious, focal cerebral symptoms
7. Headache	Moderate
8. Vomiting	Repeated
9. Meningeal symptoms	develop late, weakly expressed
10. Encephalitic symptoms	hemiparesis and convulsions, often VII, III, IV couples CN
11. Changes detected outside the nervous system	-Hemorrhagic rash -developmental pneumonia -osteomyelitis -bearing of joints -increase of liver and kidneys
12. Early complication	acute cerebral edema
13. Likvor	turbid, cytosis from 0.2 ☐ 10 / 9l to 13 ☐ 10 / 9l-in the early days of lymphocytic disease, as well as neutrophilic; unsharp increase in protein to 1g / l -Bacterium-Hemophilic rod type B -Sitting from CSF-the same
14. Blood	first, leukocytosis with a left shift and a sharp increase in ESR, later-neutrophilia with normal

	leukocyte count
15. Techenie	- Sluggish, wavy

Tuberculous meningitis

1. Epidemiological features	secondary predominantly children
2. Transmission Path	hematogenous, lymphogenic
3. Prodomal period	-long
4. Development	- sub-construction
5. Body temperature	-37-38, only towards the end it rises sharply
6. Primary symptoms	-negenialny syndrome is not clearly expressed
7. Headache	- increases by the end of the 1st week
8. Vomiting	- occurs after the rise in body temperature
9. Meningeal symptoms	- appear by the end of the first week
10. Encephalitic symptoms	-induced in the second week, after the defeat of II. III pair of CN, in the form of stunning, uncritical attitude, lack of orientation accuracy, convulsions, increased reflexes and periosteal reflexes, sometimes anisoreflexia, pathological reflexes
11. Vegetative-vascular disorders	-expressed by the end of the first week
12. Changes detected outside the nervous system	-milliary tuberculosis or focal tuberculosis of an individual organ
13. Likvor	- xanthochromia, increase in pressure, increase in protein up to 20 g / l, lymphocytic pleocytosis, a sharp decrease in sugar to 1 / 5-1 / 6 of the concentration in the blood, a sharp decrease in chloride, fibrin film after 12-24 hours - bacteriological study - Koch's wand
14. Blood	-small lymphocytic leukocytosis
15. Duration of the disease	-6-8 months

| 16. Expenditure | recovery in 75-95% of cases |

Meningitis of enterovirus etiology

1. Epidemiological features	-year-autumn period - Significant contagiousness and distinct focality - the presence of large epidemic outbreaks Preschoolers and schoolchildren are more often ill
2. Transmission Path	- air-dropping; fecal-oral
3. The period of incubation	2-7 days
4. Body temperature	- more often low-about 38; duration up to 3 days, rarely longer; in 15-20% of patients with a two-wave rise in temperature
5. Primary symptoms	- intracranial hypertension
6. Headache	-sharp short
7. Vomiting	Initially, it is frequent multiple; fast-terminating
8. Meningal symptoms	-expressed, dissociated, short-term
9. Encephalitic symptoms	- individual focal symptoms in 1/3-1/2 cases; meningoencephalitis in isolated cases
10. Likvor	- lymphocytic, sometimes neutrophilic lymphocytic pleocytosis (0.05 ... 0.5) ☐10☐9 / l, protein content normal or decreased; normalization after 14-21 days

Meningitis of mumps etiology

1. Epidemiological features	-winter-spring period - an increase in the period of epidemic diseases of the disease with parotitis - presence of contact with sick mumps Preschoolers and schoolchildren are more often ill
2. Transmission Path	- air-dropping;
3. The period of incubation	2-3 weeks
4. Body temperature	- low-grade or high, for 4-6 days; sometimes long subfebrile condition
5. Primary symptoms	- intracranial hypertension, moderately expressed meningeal symptoms
6. Headache	-strong, lasting 3-4 days

7. Vomiting	Initially, it is frequent multiple; usually no longer than 2-3 days
8. Meningeal symptoms	- in the majority of patients moderately expressed
9. Encephalitic symptoms	-separate symptoms in 50% of patients, expressed meningoencephalitis in 50% of cases
10. Likvor	- lymphocytic or mixed cytosis - (0,1 ... 1) 10^9 / l; the protein content is normal or moderately elevated; normalization after 3 weeks

Lymphocytic choriomeningitis

1. Epidemiological features	- Sporadic diseases; often small flares, more often in the spring
2. Transmission Path	- transmissible, drip, alimentary
3. The period of incubation	2-14 days
4. Body temperature	- high follow-up long subfebrile condition, sometimes undulating
5. Primary symptoms	- pronounced meningeal and hypertensive syndromes
6. Headache	-strong, initially constant, then paroxysmal
7. Vomiting	-For several days, multiple, then with attacks of headache
8. Meningeal symptoms	- sharply expressed; lasting 1-2 weeks
9. Encephalitic symptoms	-transient anisoreflexia, pyramidal signs, coordination disorders
10. Likvor	- high cytosis - (0,1 ... 1,3) 10^9 / l with a sharp prevalence of lymphocytes (80-90%), a moderate increase in protein; normalization at 3-4 weeks

Syphilitic meningitis

1. Epidemiological features	- develops in the secondary stage of syphilis, rarely in the primary and secondary. - almost exclusively in adults
2. Transmission Path	-sexual
3. The period of incubation	Absent
4. Development	-low
5. Body temperature	-do not usually go up
6. Primary symptoms	- very mildly expressed meningeal syndrome

7. Headache	- expressed
8. Vomiting	- measured
9. Meningeal symptoms	- mildly expressed
10. Encephalitic symptoms	- weak focal symptoms, often defeat II, III, VII, VIII pairs of CN
11. Changes detected outside the nervous system	- Visceral, bony or cutaneous manifestations of syphilis
12. Complications	- persistent deafness - hydrocephalus - meningomyelitis
13. Likvor	- lymphocytic pleocytosis does not exceed (0.15 - 1.5) $\cdot 10^9$ / l, sugar and chlorides are normal, the protein does not exceed 1-2 g / l, -Serological study: (+) RIBT; REEF:
14. Blood	- (+) Wassermann reaction, RIF, RIBT.
15. Duration of the disease	depends on treatment
16. Expenditure	-Experience with recovery

Dependence of the etiology of bacterial meningitis from the age of patients and the premorbid background

Predisposing factor	**Probable pathogens**
Age	
0-4 weeks	S. agalactiae, E. coli, L. monocytogenes, K. pneumoniae, Enterococcus spp., Salmonella spp.
4-12 weeks.	E. coli, L. monocytogenes, H. influenzae, S. pneumoniae, N. meningitides
3 months to 5 years	H. influenzae, S. pneumoniae, N. meningitides
5-50 years old	S. pneumoniae, N. meningitides
> 50 years	S. pneumoniae, N. meningitidis, L. monocytogenes, Enterobacteriaceae
Immunosuppression	S. pneumoniae, N. meningitidis, L. monocytogenes, Enterobacteriaceae, P. aeruginosa

Fracture of base of skull	S. pneumoniae, H. influenzae, S. pyogenes
Head trauma, neurosurgical operations and craniotomy	S. aureus, S. epidermidis, Enterobacteriaceae, P. aeruginosa
Cerebrospinal bypass	S. epidermidis, S. aureus, Enterobacteriaceae, P. aeruginosa, P. acnes
Sepsis	S. aureus, Enterococcus spp., Enterobacteriaceae, P. aeruginosa, S. pneumonia

Empirical antibacterial therapy of bacterial meningitis

Predisposing factor	**Antibiotic**
Age	
0-4 weeks	Ampicillin + cefotaxime or ampicillin + gentamicin
4-12 weeks	Ampicillin + cefotaxime or ceftriaxone
3 month.-5 year	Cefotaxime or ceftriaxone and ampicillin + chloramphenicol
5-50 year	Cefotaxime or ceftriaxone (+ ampicillin for suspected listeria), benzylpenicillin, chloramphenicol
>50 year	Ampicillin + cefotaxime or ceftriaxone
Immunosuppression	Vancomycin + ampicillin + ceftazidime
Fracture of base of skull	Cefotaxime or ceftriaxone
Head trauma, condition after neurosurgical operations	Oxacillin + ceftazidime, vancomycin + ceftazidime
Cerebrospinal bypass	Oxacillin + ceftazidime, vancomycin + ceftazidime

Antibacterial therapy of bacterial meningitis of established etiologyых

Predisposing factor	**Drugs of choice**	Alternative drugs
H. influenzae		
beta-lactamase (-)	Ampicillin	Cefotaxime, ceftriaxone, cefepime, chloramphenicol
beta-lactamase (+)	Cefotaxime or ceftriaxone	Cefepime, chloramphenicol,

		aztreonam, pefloxacin
N. meningitidis Penicillin MPC <0.1 mg / L MPC of penicillin 0.1 - 1.0 mg / l	Benzylpenicillin and ampicillin Cefotaxime or ceftriaxone Tsefmetazol, cefpir., Cefoxitin	Cefotaxime, ceftriaxone, chloramphenicol Chloramphenicol, fluoroquinolones meropenem
S. pneumoniae Penicillin MPC <0.1 mg / L MPC of penicillin 0.1 - 1.0 mg / l MPC of penicillin> 2.0 mg / l	Benzylpenicillin or ampicillin Cefotaxime or ceftriaxone Vancomycin + cefotaxime or ceftriaxone (±rifampicin) Cefmethazole with cefpyr, cefoxithem	Cefotaxime, ceftriaxone, chloramphenicol, vancomycin Meropenem, vancomycin, rifampicin
Enterobacteriaceae	Cefotaxime or ceftriaxone	Azrethra, fluoroquinolones, cotrimoxazole, meropenem
P. aeruginosa	Ceftazidime (±amikacin)	Ciprofloxacin, meropenem, aztreonam (±aminoglycosides)
L. monocytogenes	Ampicillin or benzylpenicillin (±gentamicin)	Co-trimoxazole
S. agalactiae	Azrethra + Vancomycin, Oxacillin + Tobramycin, Ampicillin or benzylpenicillin (±aminoglycosides) Rifampicin, co-trimoxazole	Cefotaxime, ceftriaxone, Vancomycin
S. aureus MSSA MRSA	Ceftazidime + Vancomycin, Oxacillin Ceftazidime + Ciprofloxacin, Meropenem	Azrethra + Vancomycin, Oxacillin + Tobramycin, Rifampicin, co-trimoxazole
S. epidermidis	Vancomycin (±rifampicin)	
Spirochetes pallidum B. burgdorferi	Benzylpenicillin Ceftriaxone or cefotaxime	Ceftriaxone, doxycycline Benzylpenicillin, Doxycycline

Daily doses of penicillin, depending on the age of the patients

Age, month.	Average weight, g	6 receptions intramuscularly, ED	Age, years	Average weight, kg	6 receptions intramuscularly, ED
Newborns	3200	1 200 000	1	10	2 400 000
1	4000	1 200 000	2	12	2 400 000
2	4800	1 200 000	3	14	2 800 000
3	5500	1 200 000	4	16	3 200 000
4	6500	1 500 000	5	17	3 400 000
5	7000	1 500 000	6	21	4 000 000
6	7500	2 000 000	7 — 9	27	2 000 000
7 — 10	8500	6 000 000	10 — 12	45	2 000 000
11 — 15	9500	9 000 000	16	-	12 000 000
			17 and older	-	24 000 000

Preparations of the group of cephalosporins used to treat bacterial meningitis

The generation of cephalosporins	A drug	Doses are single, adult intravenous or intramuscular, g	Number of administrations per day	Admission to the CSF:% liquor / serum
II	Cefuroxime	1,5	3-4	16-58
III	Ceftriaxone	2	1	14-17
	Cefotaxime	2	2-3	6-27
	Ceftazidime	2	3	28-40
IV	Tsefpyrom	2	2	4-87

Doses of antibiotics for the treatment of CNS infections in adults

Adrug	Daily dose (in / in)	Intervals between administrations (h)
Azrethon	6-8 grams	6-8
Amikacin	15-20 mg / kg	12
Ampicillin	12 grams	4
Benzylpenicillin	18-24 million units	4
Vankomitsi	2 grams	6-12
Gentamicin	5 mg / kg	8

Co-trimoxazole	10-20 mg / kg (with trimethoprim)	6-12
Meropenem	4 grams	6
Metronidazole	1.5-2 g	8
Oxacillin	9-12 g	4
Rifampicin	600 mg	24
Tobramycin	5 mg / kg	8
Chloramphenicol	4 grams	6
Cefemetazole	1-2 g	2
Cefotaxime	12 grams	6
Tsefpyrom	2 grams	2
Ceftazidime	6 grams	8
Ceftriaxone	4 grams	12-24
Ciprofloxacin	1.2 g	12

Penetration of antibacterial drugs through the BBB

Good	Good only with inflammation	Bad even with inflammation	Do not penetrate
Isoniazid	Azrethon	Gentamicin	Clindamycin
Co-trimoxazole	Azlocillin	Carbenicillin	Lincomycin
Pefloxacin	Amikacin	Lomefloxacin	
Rifampicin	Amoxicillin	Macrolides	
Chloramphenicol	Ampicillin	Norfloxacin	
	Vancomycin	Streptomycin	
	Meropenem		
	Ofloxacin		
	Benzylpenicillin		
	Cephalosporins III-IV Generations		
	Cefuroxime		
	Ciprofloxacin		

Empirical starting antibiotic therapy of bacterial meningitis depending on the clinical situation

Age up to 3 months	
Probable pathogen	N. meningitides, Hib, S. pneumoniae, E. coli, S. agalactiae, K. pneumoniae, Enterococcus spp., Listeria идр.
Drugs of choice	Chloramphenicol + Ampicillin
Alternative drugs	Cefotaxime
	Ceftriaxone
	Ampicillin + Amcacine
Age from 3 months to 6 years	
Probable pathogen	Hib, N. meningitides, S. pneumonia
Drugs of choice	Cefotaxime
	Ceftriaxone
Alternatives to Ampicillin + Amcacine	
Age from 6 to 60 years	
Probable pathogen	N. meningitides, S. pneumoniae, Hib
Drugs of choice	Penicillin
Alternative drugs	Ceftriaxone or Cefotaxime
	Meropenem
Age over 60 years	
Probable pathogen	N. meningitides, S. pneumoniae, Hib, Enterococcus spp., Listeria, Enterobacteriaceae идр.
Drugs of choice	Cephalosporins of III and IV generations
Alternative drugs	Ampicillin + Amcacine
Patients with immunodeficiency states	
Probable pathogen	S. pneumoniae, S. aureus, Listeria, Enterococcus spp., Enterobacteriaceae
Drugs of choice	CA III + Ampicillin
Alternative drugs	Ampicillin + Amcacine
	Meropenem or Vancomycin
Meningitis in the background of angioed sepsis (drug addicts)	
Probable pathogen	S. aureus, epidermidis, Enterococcus spp., Enterobacteriaceae идр.

Drugs of choice	Rifampicin + Gentamicin Ampicillin / Sulbactam + Oxacillin (daily dose of oxacillin not less than 16 g)
Alternative drugs	CA III + Amicacin or Meropenem Vancomycin + Amicacin
On a background of a septic endocarditis	
Probable pathogen	S. aureus, Staphylococcus spp. Enterococcus spp идр.
Drugs of choice	Ampicillin + Gentamicin Ampicillin / Sulbactam + Oxacillin (daily dose of oxacillin not less than 16 g)
Alternative drugs	Vancomycin + Amicacin CA III + Amicacin + Rifampicin
Neurosurgical pathology	
Probable pathogen	S. pneumoniae, S. aureus, Hib, Streptococcus spp., Staphylococcus spp., Enterococcus spp., P. aeruginosa
Drugs of choice	Ceftazidime + Vancomycin Meropenem
Alternative drugs	Oxacillin + Tobramycin Aztreon + Vancomycin
Oxacillin + Tobramycin Aztreon + Vancomycin	
Probable pathogen	S. pneumoniae, S. aureus, Hib, Streptococcus spp., Staphylococcus spp., Enterococcus spp., K. pneumonia
Drugs of choice	Ceftazidime + FX (fluoroquinolones) Meropenem Rifampicin + Co-trimoxazole
Alternative drugs	Oxacillin + Tobramycin Aztreon + Vancomycin
Rhinogenic and sinusogenic meningitis	

Probable pathogen	S. pneumoniae, S. aureus, Hib, Streptococcus spp., Staphylococcus spp., Enterococcus spp., P. aeruginosa
Drugs of choice	Ceftazidime + Vancomycin Meropenem
Alternative drugs	Oxacillin + Tobramycin Aztreon + Vancomycin
Otogenic meningitis	
Probable pathogen	S. pneumoniae, S. aureus, Hib, Streptococcus spp., Staphylococcus spp., Enterococcus spp., P. aeruginosa
Drugs of choice	Ceftazidime Ceftazidime + Vancomycin Meropenem
Alternative drugs	Oxacillin + Tobramycin Aztreon + Vancomycin
Meningitis in the background of osteomyelitis	
Probable pathogen	S. pneumoniae, S. aureus, Hib, Streptococcusspp., Staphylococcusspp., Enterococcusspp., P. aeruginosa, реже – анаэробы
Drugs of choice	CC III + FH Ceftazidime + Vancomycin
Alternative drugs	Oxacillin + Tobramycin CA III + Vancomycin Meropenem
Purulent meningitis in HIV-infected or AIDS patients	
Probable pathogen	Different gram + and gram-bacteria
Drugs of choice	CC III + FH Ceftazidime + Vancomycin The same + Co-trimoxazole
Alternative drugs	Oxacillin + Tobramycin CA III + Vancomycin Meropenem + Amikacin

Meningitis in the background of prolonged mechanical ventilation, including nosocomial	
Probable pathogen	S. pneumoniae, S. aureus, Hib, Streptococcuspp., Staphylococcusp., Enterococcuspp., P. aeruginosa, less often anaerobes, Enterobacteriaceae
Drugs of choice	Ceftazidime + Vancomycin Ampicillin + Oxacillin + Gentamicin Ceftazidime + FH Meropenem
Alternative drugs	Oxacillin + Tobramycin Aztreon + Vancomycin
Abscess of the brain	
Probable pathogen	Anaerobes, Streptococcus spp., S. aureus, Enterobacteriaceae
Drugs of choice	CS III + FX + Metranidazole CA III + Vancomycin + Metronidazole Chloramphenicol + Metronidazole
Alternative drugs	Meropenem Meropenem + Amikacin Rifampicin + Co-trimoxazole

Differential diagnosis of meningitis in the prehospital stage

Clinical form	Common complaints	The characteristic beginning	Severity of meningeal symptoms	Common infectious symptoms	Changes in consciousness
Purulent (meningococcal, pneumococcal, staphylo-streptococcal, etc.) meningitis	Rapidly growing headache, nausea, chills, vomiting	Sharp. A short continuation (several hours) is possible	Sharp with an increase in the first hours and days	A significant increase in temperature (39-40°C) chills, skin hyperemia	Stunned, sopor, coma. Sometimes delirium, hallucinations
Serous viral meningitis (mumps, enterovirus, acute lymphocytic charyomeningitis, etc.)	Headache, chills, nausea, less frequent vomiting	Acute, sometimes after catarrh of the airways and gastrointestinal disorders	Moderate, sometimes biphasic, intracranial hypertension predominates	Moderate fever, sometimes biphasic, transient (3-7 days).	Usually somnolence, less often deafness, sopor, delirium
Tuberculous meningitis	Fatigue, anorexia, sweating, nausea, mild headache	Gradual with common symptoms of asthenia, sometimes in adults acute	Minor at first with a gradual increase	Subfebrile condition with predominance of signs of intoxication	Consciousness is preserved, broken in the unfavorable course
Meningitis in general infections and somatic diseases	A slight headache	Different	Moderate	Depends on the underlying disease	No. Exception is extremely heavy forms

Differential diagnosis of purulent meningitis (meningoencephalitis) from subarachnoid hemorrhage

Reliable differential diagnostic signs

Diagnostic signs	Purulent meningitis (meningoencephalitis)	Subarachnoid haemorrhage
Results of CT or MRI	Multiple small foci of hypo-intensity. Signs of OM-constriction of subarachnoid space, interlobar fissures, ventricular system of the brain.	Areas of hyperintensity in the compartments of the subarachnoid space filled with blood.
Results of the CSF study	Purulent CSF. Severe pleocytosis with predominance of neutrophils. Sometimes protein-cell dissociation.	Bloody CSF for 1-2 days, xanthochromia in the future.

Additional differential diagnostic signs

Diagnostic signs	Purulent meningitis (meningoencephalitis)	Subarachnoid haemorrhage
Presence of background disease	Usually	Not typical, hypertensive disease possible
Onset of disease	Within hours	The sharpest, minute
Body temperature	39-40	At first, normal, then subfebrile
Consciousness	Within 12-18 hours a complete loss is possible	Not changed or short-term loss
Meningeal symptoms	Are sharply expressed except for extremely heavy current	Expressed slightly
Hemogram	Severe neutrophilic leukocytosis, increased ESR	Unchanged or unsharply changed

Differential diagnosis of purulent meningitis from an acutely manifesting abscess of the brain

Symptoms	Purulent meningitis	Acutely manifesting abscess of the brain
Results of CT or MRI	Multiple small foci of hypo-intensity. Signs of OM - narrowing of the subarachnoid space, interlobar fissures, ventricular system of the brain.	Ring-shaped hyperintensity, corresponding to the zone of perifocal edema, hypo-intensity in the area of the capsule of the abscess. Signs of generalized edema. A dislocation of the median structures is possible.
Onset of disease	Sharp, sharp	Gradually. May be preceded by inflammatory diseases of the ENT organs, pneumonia, changes in the psyche, gaol pain, changes in gait.
Consciousness	Rapid loss to soporus and coma.	Uneven gradual depression of consciousness. Sometimes a change of consciousness.
Meningeal symptoms	Are sharply expressed except for extremely heavy current	Moderately expressed
Ocular fundus	As a rule, not changed	Often, edema of the optic discs
Results of the CSF study	Purulent CSF. Severe pleocytosis with predominance of neutrophils. Sometimes protein-cell dissociation.	Moderate pleocytosis (100-300 cells per 1 µl). Often, protein-cell dissociation.
Echoencephaloscopy	The median structures of the brain are not displaced.	A displacement of the middle struts of the brain can be detected.

Encephalitis

Encephalitis is a group of diseases characterized by inflammation of the brain. Encephalitis is divided into primary and secondary, viral and microbial, infectious-allergic, allergic and toxic.

Classification

Encephalitis caused by neurotropic viruses is characteristic of epidemic, contagious, seasonal and climatic geographic features of distribution. By prevalence of pathological of the process, encephalitis with a predominant lesion of white matter is isolated - leukoencephalitis, encephalitis with predominance of lesions gray matter – polioencephalitis. Encephalitis with diffuse lesion of nerve cells and conducting brain pathways – panencephalitis. Depending on the primary localization encephalitis is divided into hemispheric, stem, cerebellar, mesencephalic, diencephalic. Often, along with the substance of the brain, some parts of the spinal cord are affected, in these cases they speak of encephalomyelitis. Encephalitis can be diffuse and focal, by the nature of the exudate – purulent and non-purulent.

Primary encephalitis	Secondary encephalitis;
• Viral:	• Viral:
• Arbovirus, seasonal, vector-borne	• with measles
• Viral without clear seasonality (polysason):	• with chicken pox
	• with rubella
• Enterovirus caused by the Coxsackie virus and ECHO	• influenza
	• Post-vaccination:
• herpetic	• DTP
• with rabies	• vaccinia vaccine
• Caused by an unknown virus:	• rabies vaccine
• epidemic (economy)	• Microbial and rickettsial:
• Microbial and rickettsial:	• staphylococcal
• with neurosyphilis	• streptococcal
• with typhus	• malarial
	• toxoplasmosis
	• Encephalitis caused by slow infections
	• subacute sclerosing panencephalitis
	• Paraneoplastic processes:
	• Anti-NMDA-receptor encephalitis (acute transient limbic encephalitis)

Clinical symptoms of encephalitis are the same for both adults and children.

The mild course of the disease:
- increased body temperature;
- nausea;
- loose stools;
- headache;
- sensitivity to light;
- epileptic seizures;
- impaired consciousness;
- drowsiness.

More severe course of the disease:
- coma;
- paralysis and paresis of limbs;
- stiff neck;
- increased number of leukocytes (in the blood);
- increased number of lymphocytes (in CSF).

Differential diagnosis of encephalitis.

Symptoms	Tick-borne encephalitis	Japanese encephalitis	Encephalitis Economome
Seasonality	Spring-summer period	Summer-autumn period	Winter-spring period
Onset of disease	Acute	Sudden	Gradual
Temperature response	Febrile - 4-6 days, can be a two-wave	Febrile 7-10 days	Subfebrile, normal
Cutaneous manifestations	Hyperemia of the face, breast	Hyperemia of the face, breast	Normal
Changes in mucous membranes	Injection sclera	Injection sclera	Normal
General cerebral symptoms	Expressed	Expressed	None
Meningeal symptoms	Expressed	Expressed	None
Changing mind and consciousness	Soporous-comatose	Soporous-comatose, delirious-amenious	Copernicus
Focal neurological symptoms	Flaccid paresis, paralysis, bulbar syndrome	Spastic paralysis, hyperkinesia, muscle rigidity	Oculomotor disorders, muscle rigidity, hyperkinesis
Blood	Leukocytosis or leukopenia	Leukocytosis or leukopenia	Not changed
Likvor		Pronounced cytosis	Unchanged or weakly expressed cytosis
Pathological and anatomical changes	Polioencephalomyelitis: lesion of spinal, stem motoneurons	Polioencephalomyelitis in the cortex, subcortical ganglia, hypothalamus	Polioencephalomyelitis in the gray matter of the midbrain, the walls of the third ventricle
Chronic forms	Kozhevnikovskaya epilepsy, other hyperkinesis, amyotrophies	Psychotic disorders	Pa-kinsonism

Primary encephalitis. Epidemic encephalitis

Criterion	Presence, manifestation
Floor	Irrelevant
Age	All age groups
Seasonality	Not typical
Etiology	Not established, epidemiological data allow to consider the causative agent of a filtering virus.
Wedge. picture: temperature	The temperature curve is usually incorrect. It rarely rises above 380.
Sleep disorders	Pathological drowsiness. Patients sleep round the clock. The dream is of an irresistible character. Insomnia is less common.
Doubling	Can stay for less than a day or for many days and weeks and is associated with paresis of the motor nerves of the eyes.
Symptom of Argyl Robertson	Back. Absence or decrease in pupil response to accommodation and convergence in the presence of a living reaction to light. Can stay for less than a day or for many days and weeks and is associated with paresis of the motor nerves of the eyes.
Vegetative disorders	Increased or decreased sweating, "sebaceous face", tachycardia, a violation of the rhythm of breathing, hypersalivation.
Ocular fundus	Mostly not modified
Paralysis and paresis of extremities	Can not be.
Sensitivity disorders	They do not.
Pathological reflexes	There are very rare
Hyperkinesis	Chorea, athetosis, myoclonia
Speech	Monotone, malovyrazitelnaya, lubricated due to muscle tone disorders
Mental disorders	They are of a kind of light excitement, accompanied by confusion and delirium. Depression is less common
Duration of acute period	From 2-4 days to 4 months.
Leukocytosis	Do not reach large numbers, polynucleated
Meningeal symptoms	Expressed slightly
Cerebrospinal fluid	Small changes: weakly positive protein reactions and small pleocytosis (up to 20 lymphocytes). Increased sugar content in the liquid

Primary encephalitis
Two-wave viral meningoencephalitis

Criteria	Availability; manifestation
Epidemiological features	There is a disease in the same natural conditions as tick-borne encephalitis. (The Far East, the Urals, Siberia)
Seasonality	July-September
The transmission path	Almentary, less often through vinegar mites
Etiology	Tick-borne encephalitis virus
The incubation period	With vinegar mite 8-20 days, with alimentary infection 4-7 days
Tick-borne encephalitis virus	Acute
With vinegar mite 8-20 days, with alimentary infection 4-7 days	Two-wave temperature curve: 5-7 days of hyperthermia, 6-10 days - remission, the second hyperthermia wave up to 10 days.
Acute	Headache, vomiting, diarrhea, constipation, congestion, puffiness of face, infection of sclerosis.
Two-wave temperature curve: 5-7 days of hyperthermia, 6-10 days - remission, the second hyperthermia wave up to 10 days.	Rigidity of the neck muscles
Headache, vomiting, diarrhea, constipation, congestion, puffiness of face, infection of sclerosis.	The changes correspond to serous meningitis.

Rigidity of the neck muscles...	Absent.
Tick-borne encephalitis virus	Sweating, thermoregulation, arterial hypotension, bradycardia, sebaceous face.
With vinegar mite 8-20 days, with alimentary infection 4-7 days	Rarely
Acute	Rarely
Two-wave temperature curve: 5-7 days of hyperthermia, 6-10 days - remission, the second hyperthermia wave up to 10 days.	Do not happen
Headache, vomiting, diarrhea, constipation, congestion, puffiness of face, infection of sclerosis.	None
Rigidity of the neck muscles...	Favorable

Primary encephalitis
Japanese encephalitis

Criterion	Availability; manifestation
Epidemiological features	Japan, Primorye Territory

Seasonality	Summer-autumn
The transmission path	Through mosquito bites
Etiology	Filtering virus from the group of arboviruses
The incubation period	10-15 days
Onset of disease	Sudden
Body temperature	A sharp rise in temperature reaches 39-41 $^\circ$ C and at this level holds 7-10 days then falls lytically.
Meningeal symptoms	Expressed
Skin covers	Hyperemic, there are multiple scattered elements of hemorrhagic rash.
Mental disorders	Psychomotor agitation, delirium, hallucinations or, on the contrary, adynamia.
Muscle tone	Increased plastic type.
Pyramidal disorders	Observed often.
Bulbar disorders	In severe cases of the disease
Peripheral parals	Seldom observed
Parkinson's Syndrome	Absent
Cerebrospinal fluid	High blood pressure, cytosis mixed, up to 200 cells per 1 mm3 protein content normal, sugar content within
Blood	Neutrophilic leukocytosis, increased ESR
Course of the disease	Extremely acute, heavy
Mortality	40-70%
Diagnostics	RSK. LV
Prevention	Dehydration of swamps, application of measures to protect against mosquitoes, use of serum convalescent or hyperimmune horse serum.

Primary encephalitis
Acute disseminated encephalomyelitis

Criterion	Presence, manifestation
Etiology	Neurotropic virus
Pathomorphology	Affected white matter of the brain and spinal cord,

	peripheral nerves, as well as the meninges. The main manifestation is multiple foci of demyelination.
The prodromal period	Short
Onset of disease	Sharp or subacute.
General cerebral symptoms	Expressed
Lesions of the cranial nerves	It occurs often. The bulbar group of cranial nerves suffer (IX, X, XII), the facial nerve, rarely the oculomotor nerves (III, IV, VI)
Movement disorders	pair - or tetraplegia. Paresis and paralysis usually develop in the legs.
Pelvic function disorders	More often a delay of urine and feces, less often incontinence.
Hyperkinesis	Seldom observed
Blood	Moderate leukocytosis, eosinophilia. ESR increased to 30-40 mm / h.
Likvor	Slight pleocytosis. A slight increase in protein content
Diagnostics	History, clinical examination and observation
Forecast	Usually favorable

Primary encephalitis.
Polysone encephalitis

Criterion	Presence, manifestation
Floor	
Age	Irrelevant
Seasonality	Children's
Etiology	Polizeason
Hemispheric syndrome	Different
Stem syndrome	Characterized by acute onset, hyperthermia, impaired consciousness convulsions, development of paralysis.
Cerebellar syndrome	It is manifested by oculomotor, vestibular, bulbar disorders.
Flow	Characteristic acute coordination disorders, ataxia, nystagmus, intentional tremor.
Cerebrospinal fluid	Not heavy

Primary encephalitis
Tick-borne encephalitis

Criterion	Presence, manifestation
Etiological features	Far East, Primorye Territory, Siberia
The transmission path	Transmissible (via vinegar mites)
Seasonality	Spring - summer
Etiology	Neurotropic virus
The incubation period	1-3 weeks
Onset of disease	Sudden
Body temperature	It rises sharply, reaching 39-400 and even 410 s
Meningeal syndrome	Expressed
Parezy and atrophic paralysis	Most often involve the muscles or the shoulder girdle and the proximal parts of the upper limbs. The "dangling" head
Bulbar paralysis	rarely
Mental disorders	Delusions of visual and auditory hallucinations, agitation or severe oppression
blood	Leukocytosis (1200-1800) was accelerated by ESR.
Likvor	Cell-protein dissociation (50-200 lymphocytes in 1 μl with a normal or slightly increased protein content) with meningeal form
Diagnostics	Complement reaction reaction neutralization reaction; hemagglutination inhibition reaction, biological experiment
Prevention	Vaccination, protection measures against vinegars and systematic destruction of forest mites

Secondary encephalitis
Measles encephalitis

Criterion	Presence, manifestation
Floor	Irrelevant
Age	Children
Etiology	Corpuscle virus
Seasonality	Not typical
Onset of disease	Acute, usually on the 3-5th day after the rash.
Temperature	By the beginning of encephalitis can normalize, and often

	notice a new sharp rise to a high level.
Consciousness	Confused
Mental disorders	Psychomotor agitation, hallucinations, delirium.
Meningeal symptoms	Expressed insignificantly
Epileptic seizures	Often observed
Parezy, Pallas	Identified by examination
Extrapyramidal symptoms	Trembling of the head and limbs, choreoathetoid, myoclonic cramps.
Symptoms of defeat of the II.III.VII cranial nerves	Often observed
Sensitivity disorders	By explorer type
Pelvic disorders	Due to the involvement of the spinal cord (measles encephalomyelitis)
Likvor	The fluid pressure is increased. Increased protein content and increased cytosis
Course of the disease	Heavy
Mortality	Up to 25%

Secondary encephalitis
Sypnotifose encephalitis

Criterion	Presence, manifestation
Etiology	The causative agent of typhus
General cerebral symptoms	Dominate over all other manifestations of the disease.
The Delusional Period	There is a trembling and support of the muscles of the face. Stereotype movements of the hands of a swallowing disorder, hyperkinesis or hemiparesis.
Cerebrospinal fluid	Increased pressure, weakly positive protein reactions, small cytosis. The liquid is clear, sometimes xanthrome. The Weil-Felix reaction and the gelolysin reaction are positive.
Complication	Myelitis (pelvic disorders spinal paresis and trophic disorders).
Exodus	Recovery
Effects	Hemiparesis, persistent hyperkinesia of cerebellar disorders.

Secondary encephalitis
Vaccinal encephalitis

Criterion	Presence, manifestation
Floor	Irrelevant
Age	In childhood, and in adults, primarily vaccinated people.
The incubation period	Not the same in different countries
Onset of disease	At 7-9-12 - the day after vaccination, the disease develops sharply.
Temperature	A sharp rise to 390-400C.
Consciousness	Dullness of consciousness, reaching to coma in severe cases.
Meningeal symptoms	Revealed rarely.
Neurological focal symptoms	Epileptiform seizures, mono- and hemiparesis, oculomotor, pupillary disorders, paresis of the facial and sublingual nerves.
Violation of the function of the pelvic organs	They are rare.
The defeat of the extrapyramidal system	Hyperkinesis, a violation of coordination of movements.
Cerebrospinal fluid	Increased pressure, small lymphocytic cytosis. The protein content is normal
Blood	There are no specific changes.
Flow and outcome	Usually favorable. In severe cases, patients fall into a coma or epileptic status and die several hours after the onset of the disease.
Diagnostics	The support for the correct diagnosis is a firmly established fact of vaccination for 7-12 days before the disease
Prevention	Timely (up to 6 months) vaccination

Secondary encephalitis
Influenza encephalitis

Criterion	Presence, manifestation
Etiology	Viruses of type A (A1A1A2) and B
Occurrence of symptoms of encephalitis	Mainly within the first week of onset of the disease; less often begin to speak later

Encephalitic symptoms	Headache, nausea, photophobia, pyramidal signs, single epileptic seizures
Meningeal symptoms	Expressed slightly
Likvor	Increased pressure, moderate amount of protein, small pleocytosis
Course of the disease	It lasts from several days to a month and ends with recovery
Mortality	Occurs in isolated cases

Secondary encephalitis
Rheumatic encephalitis

Criterion	Presence, manifestation
Frequency of occurrence of the disease	Very rare form
Etiology	β- hemolytic streptococcus type A.
Temperature	Increases to 37.5-39 0C, the temperature curve is incorrect
Headache	Excruciating
Vomiting	It happens often
Skin and mucous membranes	Pale
Focal Symptoms	Mono- and hemiparesis, lesion of craniocerebral nerves, cortical, stem, diencephalic, capsular or striatal syndromes
Epileptic seizures	Jacksonian, general
Changes of mind	Occurs quite often
Likvor	The pressure is increased, the color is transparent. The amount of protein is increased, pleocytosis reaches 100-150, rarely to higher digits.
Course of the disease	Very heavy
Exodus	Mortality or severe disability
Diagnostics	Anamnesis, an indication of rheumatism in the past, characteristic changes in the heart, elevated ESR, positive immunobiochemical tests for rheumatism (C-reactive protein, diphenylalanine test, increased transaminase level)
Prevention	Primary and secondary prevention of rheumatism

Secondary encephalitis
Encephalitis in chicken pox

Criterion	Presence, manifestation
Floor	Irrelevant
Age	Children's
Etiology	Viral
Onset of disease	Fast - 3-7 days after the appearance of rashes
Temperature	Hyperthermia
Meningeal symptoms	Positive
Consciousness	Comatose
Epileptic seizures	There are rarely
Pyramid violations	Observed often
Extrapyramidal disorders	Revealed often
Signs of cerebral edema	Appear early
Cerebrospinal fluid	The pressure is increased, increased protein and cytosis, the number of cells does not exceed 100-200 in 1 µl
Flow and outcome	Usually favorable

Early neurological manifestations of HIV infection
Toxoplasmic encephalitis

Criterion	Presence, manifestation
Etiology	Toxoplasma
Onset of disease	Sharp, subacute
Focal Symptoms	Are sharply expressed: mono- and hemiparesis, aphasia, hemianopsia, extrapyramidal disorders.
Epileptic seizures	Jacksonian, general
Meningeal symptoms	Absent or not clearly expressed
Likvor	An abrupt lymphocytic pleocytosis (less than 100 cells per 1 µl), a slight increase in protein and glucose.
CT or MRI	Multiple small foci of increased density and large foci of heterogeneous structure
Exodus	Mortality in 25-30%

Treatment of encephalitis

Etiotropic therapy. Etiotropic therapy consists in the appointment of a homologous gamma globulin titrated against tick-borne encephalitis virus. Gamma-globulin is recommended to inject 6 ml intramuscularly, daily for 3 days. In addition, serum immunoglobulin and homologous polyglobulin are used, which are obtained from the blood plasma of donors living in natural foci of tick-borne encephalitis. In the first day of treatment, serum immunoglobulin is recommended to be administered 2 times at intervals of 10-2 h for 3 ml with a light course, 6 ml each for moderate and 12 ml for severe. In the next 2 days, the drug is prescribed 3 ml once intramuscularly. Homologous polyglobulin is administered intravenously for 60-00 ml.

Antiviral drugs.

With pronounced phenomena of intoxication, infusion therapy is performed. With edema of the brain, bulbar disorders, the fastest effect is intravenous administration of prednisolone (2 mg / kg) or dexazone, hydrocortisone. With agitation seizures intravenously or intramuscularly injected seduksen -0,3-0,4 mg / kg of sodium oxybutyrate - 50-100 mg / kg, droperidol - from 0.5 to 8.6 ml, hexenal - 10% solution 0.5 ml / kg (with preliminary administration of atropine); enemas - chloral hydrate 2% solution of 50-100 ml.Dlya dehydration and control brain swelling and edema using 10-20% mannitol solution at 1-1.5 g / kg intravenously; L-lysine aescinat 0.1% -10 0 IV, furosemide 20-40 mg intravenously or intramuscularly, 30% glycerol 1-1.5 g / kg orally.

- Antihistamine
- Antipyretic drugs
- Anti-inflammatory
- Anticonvulsant therapy (benzonale, diphenin, finlepsin)
- Disintoxication therapy (saline solutions, protein preparations, plasma substitutes)
- Resuscitative measures (ventilation, cardiotropic drugs)
- Prevention of secondary bacterial complications (wide-spectrum antibiotics)

Restorative treatment. After discharge from the hospital in the presence of neurologic disorders, restorative treatment is carried out-neuroprotective, vasoactive drugs, B vitamins, immunocorrective therapy.

Treatment of Parkinsonism. An effective method of treatment of parkinsonism is the use of L-DOPA (a precursor of dopamine). The drug penetrates the blood-brain barrier and compensates for the lack of dopamine in the basal ganglia.

Treatment of hyperkinesia. Assign metabolic drugs, α-adrenoblockers, neuroleptics (haloperidol, aminazine) and tranquilizers.

Treatment of Kozhevnikovskaya epilepsy. Also prescribed metabolic drugs, anticonvulsants, tranquilizers and neuroleptics.

Crainocerebral trauma. Classification

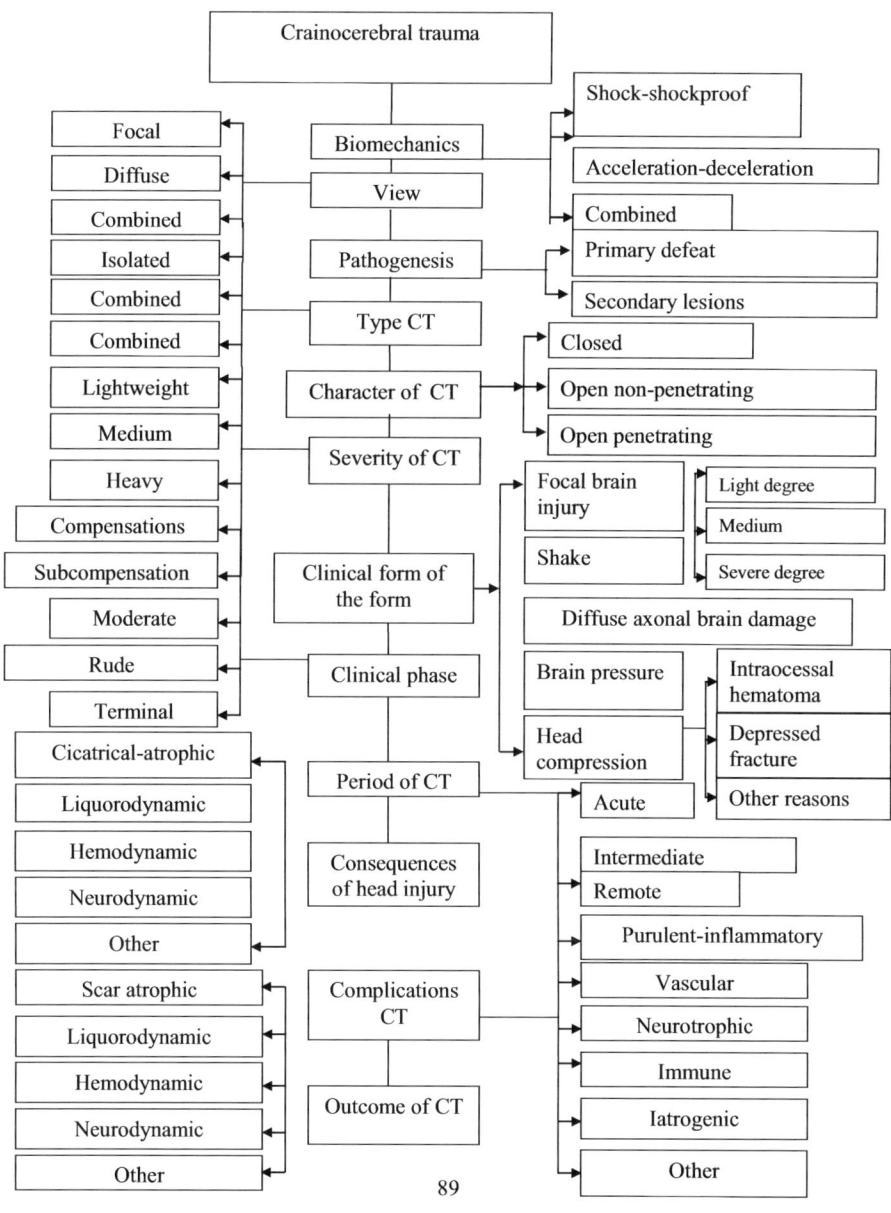

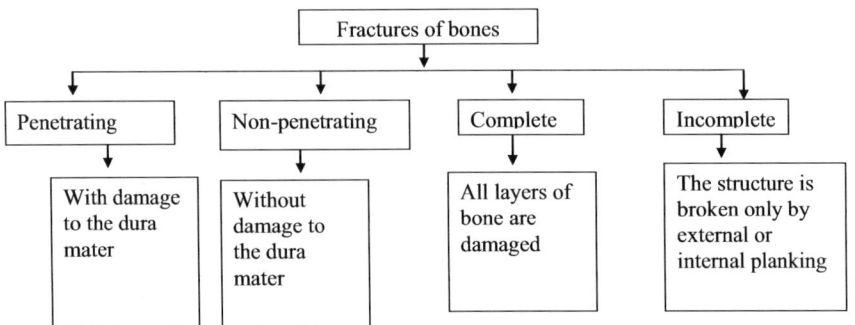

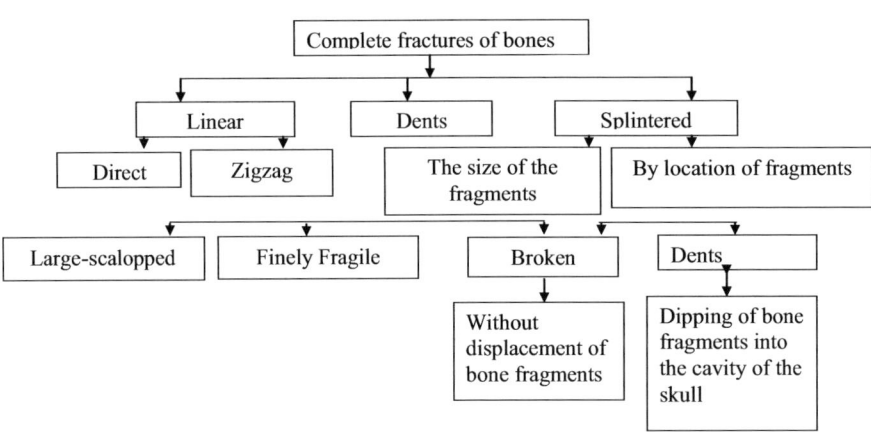

Focal neurological disorders

The level is struck	Manifestations of signs	Characteristics of lesions
The trunk of the brain (stem signs)	a) are not detected	No anisocoria, corneal reflexes are caused, there is no nystagmus, a living reaction of pupils to light;
	b) the initial	Corneal reflexes are reduced from one or both sides, clonic spontaneous nystagmus, insignificant anisocoria;
	c) expressed	Strong anisocoria, clono- tonic nystagmus, a decrease in the response of pupils to light from one or both sides. Moderate paresis of the gaze upward; Bilateral pathological signs;
	d) rough	Coarse anisocoria, coarse paresis of the gaze upward, tonic multiple spontaneous nystagmus or a floating gaze, coarse divergence of the eyeballs along the horizontal or vertical axis, rough bilateral pathological signs, extensor convulsions; Bilateral mydriasis without pupillary reaction to light, areflexia, muscle atony;
The hemisphere (hemi- and cranioblastic symptoms)	a) are not detected	Tendon and skin reflexes are normal on both sides, there are no pathological reflexes and paresis of the limbs;
	b) the initial	Decrease in abdominal reflexes (or they are not caused), unilateral increase of tendon reflexes, moderate pathological reflexes on the one hand, "soft" mono or hemiparesis, "soft" speech disorders
	c) expressed	
	d) rough	Pronounced mono- or hemiparesis, paresis of cranial nerves, speech disorders, paroxysmyclonic or clonicotonic convulsions in the extremities.
	e) Critical	Coarse mono-or hemiparesis or paralysis, verbal disorders, often recurrent clonotonic convulsions in the limbs Triparaz, triplegia, tetraparesis, tetraplegia, bilateral paresis of the facial nerve, total aphasia, constant convulsions in the limbs.

Organization of medical care

Doctor's tasks at the prehospital stage:
1. Pre-hospital examination of the patient, assessment of the state of vital functions.
2. Provide the necessary amount of medical care.
3. The fastest delivery to a specialized hospital.

Duration of acute and intermediate period of CCI

Clinical forms of trauma	Periods	
	Acute (weeks)	Intermediate (months)
1Shake	1-2	2
2. Bruising: Easy Average Heavy	2-3 4-5 6-8	2 4 6
3.Diffuse axonal injury	8-10	6
4. Pressures: Acute Podystroie Chronic	8-10 3-8 (depending on the background)	6 6 4

The severity of CT

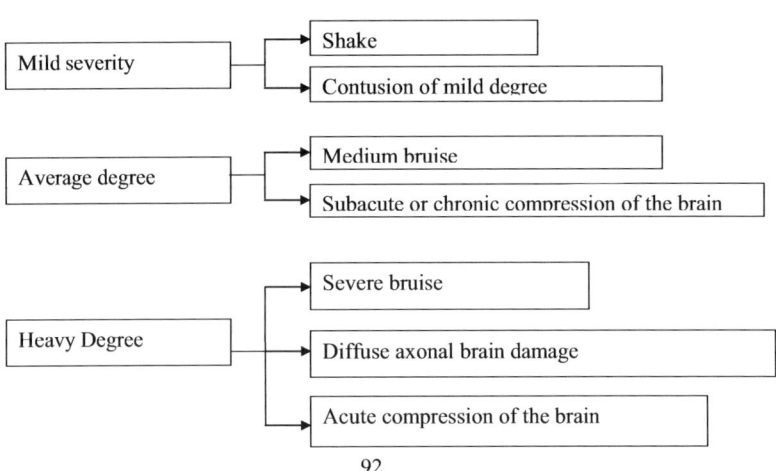

Determination of the severity of patients with craniocerebral trauma.

Degrees	The condition of the victim	Unified criteria for the severity of the condition (violations were given for each feature)			
		Consciousness	Vital functions	Focal Symptoms	
				Secondary	Primary
1	Satisfactory	Clear	No violations	No	No or mildly expressed
2	Moderate Gravity	Clear or moderate stunning	No violations (only brady is possible cardia)	-	There are various hemispheres and craniobasal symptoms, more often elective
3	Heavy	Deep stun or snuff	Disrupted predominantly moderately for 1-2 signs	Single is mildly expressed	There are gross hemispheric and craniobasal irritations and prolapses
4	Extremely heavy	Moderate or deep coma	Roughly violated on several grounds	Expressed clearly, often tentorial level	Coarse hemispheric, craniobasal and stem
5	Terminal	Beyond Limit	Catastrophic state	Ultimate mydriasis	Overlapping of cerebral and trunks. violated.

Conservative treatment of TBI

Tasks:
1. Correction of hemostasis
2. Correction of energy exchange
3. Adequate breathing
4. Recovering the CAS function
5. Stabilization of cell membranes

6. Maintenance of microcirculation in the brain
7. Prevention of hypoxia, ischemia, edema and dislocation of the brain

Treatment of lung TBI

Bed rest for 1 week
- To relieve pain - taking analgesics
- To relieve anxiety, tension and sleep disorders, sedatives, anxiolytics, antidepressants
- Desensitizing agents
- Wegetotropona means
- Means that improve microcirculation and restore vascular tone
- Capillary stabilizing agents (L-lysine escinate)
- Dehydrating agents
- Neuroprotective and normalizing metabolism of neurotransmitters
- Remedies for vascular permeability

Inpatient treatment for 7-10 days

Treatment of moderate to severe TBT

Basic goals:
- Fighting hypoxia and brain ischemia.
- Improvement of energy supply to the brain and its blood flow.
- Reduced cerebral edema and high blood pressure.
- Restoration of the blood-brain barrier.
- Prevention and elimination of inflammatory processes.
- Normalization of metabolism.
- Early rehabilitation (rehabilitation) therapy.

The whole therapy is aimed at preserving, and in the future, restoring the vital activity of the brain cells around the focus of the injury.

Inpatient treatment on average 3 weeks.
Improvement of rheological properties of blood:
Means for improving energy supply to brain tissue:
- Antioxidants
- Antihypoxants
- Means that improve cerebral blood flow
- Neuroprotective

Adequate dehydration therapy:
- Hormonal preparations.
- Anesthetics.

With subarachnoid hemorrhages:
- Antienzymes
- Anti-inflammatory drugs
- Preventing seizures (carbamazepine for 6-12 months)

The main groups of drugs used for TBI.

Drug Groups	Preparations, doses, methods of administration	Duration
1. Antihypoxants - activators of the electrotransport system of mitochondria	Cytochrome C: 50-80 mg / day. (in 200.0 ml of a 0.9% solution of NaCl) - Riboxin: up to 400 mg / day (+ 0.9 NaCl-200-250 ml) -Oxibutyrate sodium: 20-30 mg / kg body weight per single administration	10-14 days 10 days
2. Antioxidants	Emoksipin: 1% solution, 10-15 mg / kg per day for 200.0 ml of 0.3% NaCl solution - α-tocopherol acetate-300-400 mg / day inside. - Diavitol-50 ml per 200.0 ml 0.9% NaCl solution	10-12 days 15 days 15 days
3. Means that reduce the volume of tissue fluid	- L-Lysine escinate -0.1% 5.0-10.0ml IV - Lasix -05-1 mg / kg per day. w / m - Mannitol -1-1.5 mg / kg per day. in / in the cap. - Albumin-10% solution 0.2-0.3 grams per 1 kg of body weight per day.	10-15 days
4. Proteolysis inhibitors	- Kontrikal (gordoks, trasilol) 100-150 thousand units per day (single dose-20-30 thousand units) in / in the cap. for 300-500 ml of a 0.9% solution of NaCl	the first 3-5 days
5. Funds normalizing the functions of the RASK system (regulating the	Trental: 0.1-0.2 g per day. on 250-500 ml. 0.9% Na Cl solution in / in cap. - Repoliglyukin: 400-500 ml per day IV caps. - Reogluman: 10 ml per 1 kg of body weight per day. in / in the cap.	4-5 days 4-5 days 4-5 days

| aggregate state of blood) | Native plasma: 100-150 ml per day
Complamine: 5-6 ml of 15% glucose solution | 4-5 days |
|---|---|---|
| 6. Means stimulating reparative processes and normalizing the exchange of neurotransmitters | - Ceraxon in / 1000mg 2 times a day
- Nootropics (nootropil, piracetam) - 1.6-2.4 g per day
- Cerebrolysin: 10-30 ml IV | 2-3 months
2-3 weeks
20-30 days |
| 7. Vitamins | - Vitamin B1: 2-3 mg / day
- Vitamin B6: 0.05-0.1 g IM
- Vitamin C: 0.1 g IM or IV | 20-30 days
15-20 days |
| 8. Means that reduce the immunological reactivity of the body and hypertension of nervous tissue | - Diprazin: 0.025 g 2-3 times w / m
- Suprastin: 0,02 g 2,3 times per day IM
- Diphenhydramine: 0.01 g 2-3 times per day IM | |
| 9. Anticonvulsants | - Carbamazepine: 0.2 g to 2-3 times a day
- Convullex: 300 mg 2-3 times a day | |
| 10. Antibiotics and hormones | - Ceftriaxone: 1 gr 1-2 times a day
- Penicillin: 6 million per day and more
- Dexamethasone: 8 - 24 mg per day | |

Treatment of severe TBI
- Pharmacotherapy.
- Resuscitative measures.
- Restorative measures.

The objectives of pharmacotherapy:
Intensive therapy to restore the function of vital organs and systems.

Pathogenetic correction of the links of disorders of the metabolism of nervous tissue:
- *control of edema of brain substance:* drugs that reduce the volume of tissue fluid, dehydrating agents
- *membrane-protector preparations*: elimination of disturbances in energy metabolism.

Correction of system function disorders that regulate the aggregate state of blood (RASK):
trental, reopolyglucin, compliance, native plasma.

Suppression of the activity of proteolytic enzymes, which appear due to the destruction of cytoplasmic membranes:
- *Inhibitors of proteolysis:* countercrital, gordoks.
- *Detoxifying agents.*

Means that reduce the damaging effect of excess catecholamines:
- Antihistamines.

Activation of reparative processes and normalization of neurotransmitter exchange:
- Ceraxon, nootropil, cerebrolysin, actovegin. Cerebrolysin.

Prevention of post-traumatic epilepsy:
- *Anticonvulsants:* **finlepsin, convulux**.

Prevention of purulent-inflammatory complications:
- Antibiotics
- Sulfonamides
- Immunocorrective agents.

Anesthesia:
- Non-narcotic analgesics
- Narcotic analgesics

Reduction of hyperthermia: inflammatory and central genesis:
- Liqueur cocktails
- Craniocerebral hypothermia.

Contusions of the brain (contusioceredri)
Areas of brain damage of varying degrees and sizes.

By degree	By localization	In the prevalence	They are accompanied by

- lungs - medium-heavy - heavy	- convective - basal departments - subcortical structures - brain stem	- local - shared - hemispheric - generalized - with crushing brain (cerebral detritus)	- Subarachnoidal hemorrhage - fracture of the fornix and base of the skull swelling and swelling of the brain changes in the ventricles and subarachnoid spaces

1. **bruised brain contusion of mild degree:**

Pathomorphology:
- the structure of the brain and soft membranes is not broken.
- on the shells small foci and groups of drain points impregnating the blood of thesurface of one or more gyri.
- local edema of the brain around damaged areas.
- more pronounced signs of concussion.

Clinic:
- loss of consciousness from a few minutes to 1 hour.
- more intense and prolonged pain.
- vomiting, often repeated.

Focal neurological disorders:
- moderate and regressive
- meningeal syndrome
- there are fractures of the skull and subarachnoid hemorrhages.

Exodus:
Favorable. The recurrence of the symptoms of the injury within 2-3 weeks.

2. **bruised brain of medium gravity:**

Pathomorphology:
- moderate hemorrhagic impregnation of the brain tissue, destroyed by trauma.
- shallow focal hemorrhage in the area of injury
- several convolutions are damaged, white matter of the brain.
- subarachnoid hemorrhage.

- fractures of the arch and base of the skull.
- local or partial perifocal edema of the brain.

Clinic:
- coarser and prolonged signs of easy bruising.
- loss of consciousness 4-6 hours
- transient brady and tachycardia
- increased blood pressure.
- subfebrile body t^0.

Stem symptoms:
- nystagmus
- dissociation of the tone, reflexes along the axis of the body

Exodus:
More often favorable. Focal symptoms disappear after 3-5 weeks or remain weakly expressed, residual effects are possible in a separated period.

a) Violation of cardiovascular activity:
1. Increased blood pressure, tachycardia, arrhythmia. It usually normalizes after elimination of respiratory function disorders.
2. Decrease in blood pressure:
   - pain shock
   - hemorrhagic shock
   - intoxication, etc.

Pre-hospital care:
- to lower the head of the patient
- indirect cardiac massage (when it stops)
- Cardiac preparations: caffeine p / k, korglikon, strofantine iv, epinephrine IV, intracardiac, ephedrine IV
- drugs to replenish the volume of circulating blood: glucose, (saline solutions, dextrans).
- hormones: with severe cardiovascular disorders.

b) Pain shock
- immobilization
- blockade of fracture sites with novocaine
• The introduction of morphine drugs is inappropriate because of the risk of respiratorydepression and obscuring neurological symptoms.

c) **Stopping of bleeding**

d) **Psychomotor agitation:** seduxen (iv, w / m). Aminazine is not administered, t. reduces symptoms of compression of the brain, dramatically reduces blood pressure.

e) **Convulsions: inhalation of nitrous oxide with air or oxygen (1: 1)**

Vascular diseases of the nervous system

Stages of medical care for patients with acute disorders of cerebral circulation

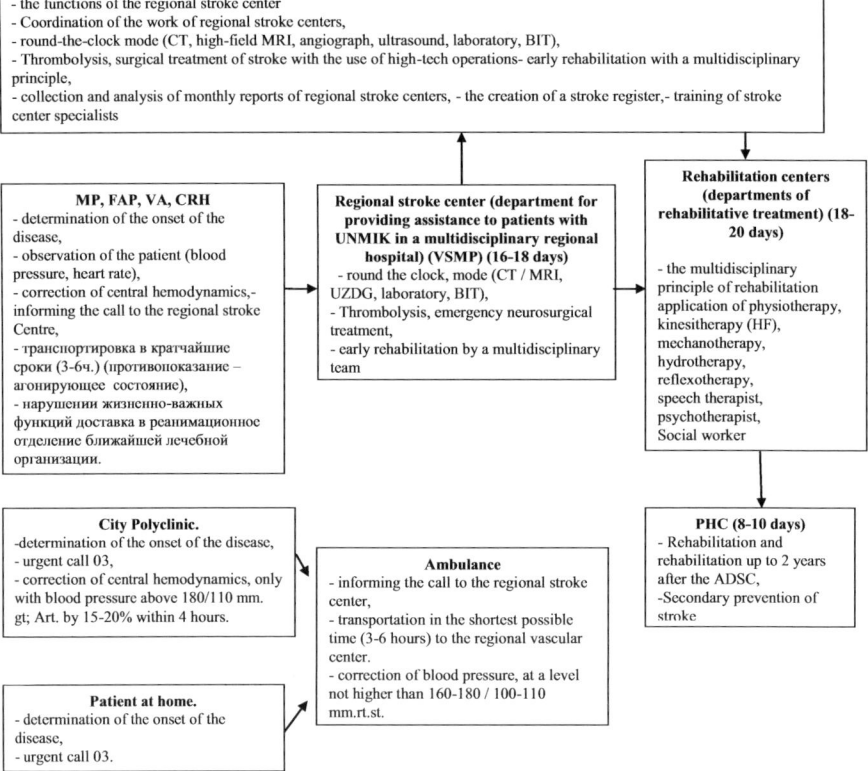

Principles of diagnosis at the admission department

Confirmation of diagnosis: CEREBRAL INSULT

1. VASCULAR ANAMNESIS (arterial hypertension, ischemic heart disease, postinfarction coronary-cardiosclerosis, rheumatism, other forms of connective tissue pathology, cardiac rhythm disturbances, vasculitis, blood diseases)

2. The appearance of neurologic symptoms on the background of paroxysmal hemodynamic disorders (fluctuations in blood pressure, cardiac rhythm disturbance, myocardial ischemia)

3. DIFFERENTIAL DIAGNOSTICS with epileptic status, trauma and brain tumors and other diseases

↓

NEURORENANIMATSIYA, DEPARTMENT OF INTENSIVE NEUROLOGY, ACUTE INSULT DIVISION
first 3-5 days

↓

1. *The first 6 hours after the development of a stroke, regardless of the severity of the patient's condition and age, the nature and localization of the process.*
2. **From 6 to 48 hours from the time of stroke:**
a. with a clear consciousness or with a disorder of consciousness before the stages of stunning-convoy-superficial coma (stage 1).
b. with a combined acute cardiac pathology (myocardial infarction, subendocardial ischemia, cardiac rhythm disturbances).
at. with decompensation of other somatic pathology (chronic kidney failure, liver).
g. in the presence of an epileptic fit in the onset.

↓

| Neuroreanimation | Department of General or Vascular Neurology | Consultation Neurosurgery |

Examination of the Sick

Specification of the character of the STROKE

In favor of ischemic stroke	In favor of hemorrhagic stroke
• A sharp decline in blood pressure below the working figures • Paroxysm of atrial fibrillation • Tachycardia • Color of face: Pale • Conjunctiva: Calm • Breath: Calm	• Increase in systemic blood pressure Above 180 for normotonics Above 200 in hypertensive patients • Bradycardia • Complexion: Bagrovacianotic • Conjunctiva: Injected • Breathing: Snoring

Examination of a patient with a diagnosis: "Acute disturbance of cerebral circulation" in the reception room

Research	Ischemic stroke	Hemorrhagic stroke
CT	in the first hours: in all cases it is possible to establish a hemorrhagic stroke, in 60% - ischemic; at the end of the first day - almost 100% of the diagnosis	
Radiography of the skull	Promotes diff. diagnosis with a tumor	promotes diff. diagnosis of herbs.
ECG	- ischemic, postinfarction changes of the myocardium - rhythm disturbances - cardiac hypertrophy	Hypertrophy of the heart
Pulse	- Reduction of pulsation of peripheral and main arteries - presence of steal syndrome	tense, often slow
Auscultation of MAG	- reveals a decrease in pulsation of carotid arteries	
AP	- pathological noises	severe arterial hypertension
Peripheral blood analysis	in severe cases - small leukocytosis and lymphopenia with Crabs index 3-5	- leukocytosis - neutrophilia with a shift to the left Crabs index above 6-7 - aneosinophilia

		- increase in hemoglobin and erythrocytes
EchoEG	The asymmetry of the median signal is possible with a slight shift towards the unaffected hemisphere	- displacement of the M-ECHO towards the unaffected hemisphere - signs of cerebral edema and intracranial hypertension - can be observed signals with limited hematoma
CF	- without pronounced changes - there may be a slight increase in protein and pressure	- bloody or xanthromic - After centriphlation, xantho-chromium is retained - flows under increased pressure - in the sediment red blood cells and macro - protein content increased

```
DIVISION OF GENERAL OR
   VASCULAR NEUROLOGY
         2-4 weeks
```

1. Hospitalization on the 3rd day of a stroke or at a later date
2. From 6 to 48 hours from the time of stroke:
   a. in the presence of deep coma.

Differential diagnostics of different types of ADSC

Differential criteria	Hemorrhagic stroke		Ischemic stroke
	Hemorrhage in the brain	*Subarachnoid haemorrhage*	*Thrombosis of the vessels of the brain*
Age	More often than 45-60 years old	More often than 20-40 years old	More often after 50
Prodromal	Can be severe	There may be	Often transient

phenomena	headache	transient vascular headaches	focal neurological symptoms
Type of patient	Hyperemia of the face, injection of the sclera	Hyperemia of the face, blepharospasm	Pallor
Onset of disease	Sudden, more often in the afternoon after physical or psychoemotional stress	Sudden, often with a sense of "blow" in the head	Gradual, more often at night, in the morning
Impairment of consciousness	Often, it quickly develops to a deep coma	Often, a short-term	Gradual development, correlates with the increase in focal symptoms
Headache	Often	Often	Rarely
Motor excitement	Often	Often	Rarely
Vomiting	70-80%	more than 50%	Rarely (2-5%)
Breath	Arrhythmic, bubbling	Often the Cheyne-Stokes rhythm may be bronchorrhea	Rarely disturbed by hemispheric foci
Pulse	Tense, brady-less often tachycardia	Increased to 80-100 per minute	Can be speeded up, soft
A heart	The boundaries are widened, the accent of the 2nd tone on the aorta	Pathological changes are rare	Often postinfarction cardiosclerosis, signs of a "hypertonic" heart
HELL	Arterial hypertension	Most often increased (may not be changed)	Can be any
Paralysis, paresis of the limbs	Hemiplegia with hyperreflexia, hormometonia	May be absent, knee reflexes are often depressed	Uneven hemiparesis, can grow to hemiplegia
Pathological symptoms	Often bilateral, more pronounced contralateral foci	Often bilateral	One-sided
Rate of development	Fast	Fast	Gradual

Convulsions	Infrequently	У 30%	Rarely
Miningeal symptoms	Often	Rarely	Rarely
Floating look	Often	Rarely	Rarely
Likvor	Bloody or xanthromic, the pressure is increased, in the sediment red blood cells and macrophages	Bloody or xanthromic, the pressure is increased, in the sediment red blood cells and macrophages	Colorless, transparent, without pronounced changes
Ocular fundus	Rarely hemorrhages, altered blood vessels	Often hemorrhages	Sclerotic changes in blood vessels
EES	The M-echo is shifted toward the unaffected hemisphere, signs of cerebral edema and intracranial hypertension, signals from a limited hematoma	M-echo is not biased, signs of cerebral edema and intracranial hypertension	M-echo, as a rule, is not displaced, there may be interhemispheric asymmetry up to 2 mm - in the first days of a stroke

ALGORITHMS OF DIAGNOSIS AND TREATMENT OF THE INSULT
Differential diagnosis of the nature of stroke
on clinical manifestations of the disease

Clinic manifestations of disease	Hemorrhagic	Ischemic	
		Non-emblematic	Embolic
Age	45-60 years old, with SAC 20-40 years old	After 50 years	Any age in the presence of a source of embolism

Pre-existing diseases	With IUD - arterial hypertension, long-lasting, with a crisis current	Symptoms of myocardial ischaemia, lower limbs	Heart Disease
Prodroma	Headache	Transient focal symptoms	No
Onset of disease	Sudden, more often in the afternoon after physical or psycho-emotional tension. With SAC - a sense of "blow" in the head.	Sudden, more often at night, in the morning, there may be a gradual increase in symptoms	Sudden
Complexion	Hyperemia	Pallor	Pallor
Conjunctiva	Injected	features	
Breath	Snoring	Most not changed	
AP	Pronounced AG	There are various options (normo-, hypo-, hypertension)	
Pulse	A strained, not-rarely bradycardia, can be tachy-cardia	Reduction of the pulse of peripheral and trunk arteries, the presence of the syndrome of stalking. There may be a tachycardia	Diseases of the heart: paroxysmal tachycardia, atrial fibrillation, etc.
Impairment of consciousness	Characteristically the oppression of consciousness rapidly aggravates to a deep coma	Gradual development, correlates with the increase of focal symptomatology	Often in the debut of the disease or can quickly develop later, correlates with the severity of focal symptomatology
Motor excitement	Often	rarely	rarely
Vomiting	70-80%	rarely (2-5%)	Often(25-30%)
Paralysis, paresis of the limbs	Hemiplegia with hyper-reflection, hormone-tonia	Uneven hemiparesis, can grow to hemiplegia	Uneven hemi-miparez, more often g-miplegia

Pathological symptoms	Often bilateral, more pronounced contralateral hearth	One-sided	More often One-sided
Convulsions	When IUD is rare, at SAK - up to 30%	Rarely	Often as a debut Diseases
Meningeal symptoms	Often, with SAK are characteristic	Rarely	Lungs
Floating look	Often	Rarely	Rarely
Vegetative-trophic violations, greasiness, sweating of the skin, paroxysmal violations muscular tone, hormone, bullous decubitus	Often, expressed	Rarely, moderately expressed	
Auscultation of MAG	Without pathology	Decreases the ripple of the carotid arteries, pathological noises	

Differential diagnosis of the nature of stroke according to additional research methods

Additional methods research	Hemorrhagic	Ischemic	
		Non-emblematic	Embolic
ECG	Hypertrophy of departments hearts	Ischemic, postinfarction changes in the myocardium, rhythm disturbances	
Ocular fundus	Hemorrhages, modified vessels	Changes in blood vessels (atherosclerosis, vasculitis, etc.)	
Echoencephaloscopy	M-echo shifted to one hundred unaffected	M-echo is usually not biased, there may be an interhemispheric asymmetry about 2 mm in the first	

	hemispheres, signs cerebral edema and intra_ cranial hypertension, may be observed bounded from hematoma	days of a stroke
Radiography skulls	Without pathology (contributes to differential diagnosis with traumatic brain injury)	
CT scan of the head brain	The first clock: in all cases allows you to install hemorrhagic Ragic character of a stroke, in 60% - ischemic; at the end of the first day - almost 100% diagnosis	
MND of the brain	It allows to obtain an image of hemorrhage and hematoma, to reveal signs of cerebral edema, blood penetration into the liquor-conducting pathways and their displacement	It allows to obtain the image of the zone of necrosis (infarction), including in the area of the trunk, to reveal the signs of perifocal edema and the displacement of the liquor-dynamic pathways. In angiographic mode, the image of the vessels is non-invasive
X-ray contrast angiography	Confirms the presence of the pathology of cerebral vessels before the planned neurosurgical intervention	
Ultrasound of the main arteries of the head, duplex **scanning, transcranial doppler**ography	Identify the presence of pathological malformations	There are atherosclerotic plaques and hemodynamically significant stenosis of the arteries, a decrease in the rate and a change in the direction of the blood flow along the extra- and intracranial vessels
TPC	Bloody or xanth-chrome, after centrifugation of xanth-chromium is preserved; it results under elevated pressure, in erythrocytes and macrophages, the protein content is increased. Can be colorless, transparent, without pronounced changes or with a slight increase in the content of protein	Colorless, transparent, without expressed changes. There may be a slight increase in protein and pressure

EEG	Reflects the presence of cerebral disorders, interhemispheric asymmetry, focal changes and the development of secondary stem syndrome. Nonspecific for the nature of the stroke	
Echocardiography	Dilation of heart cavities and hypertrophy of the walls of the heart	Signs of the pathology of the myocardium, heart pockets, presence of thrombi or mi-xome in the cavities and valves of the heart
Hemocoagulation	In the acute period, a more characteristic increase in fibrinolytic activity	In the acute period is more characteristic reduction of bleeding time and blood coagulation, increase in fibrinogen, prothrombin, increase of plasma tolerance to hepatitis, change of APTT (activated partial thromboplasty time), increase of adhesion and aggregation of platelets, decreased elasticity of erythrocyte membranes
Analysis peripheral blood	Leukocytosis, neutrophilia with a shift to the left, aneosinophilia, elevation of hemoglobin and erythrocytes	in severe cases - a small leukocytosis and lymphopenia

Classification of intracerebral hemorrhages depending on the location in relation to the inner capsule and brain areas

1. Supratentorial:
    - medial (thalamic) - medial than the inner capsule;
    - lateral (putamenal) - lateral than the inner capsule;
    - subcortical (lobar) - close to the cortex of the large hemispheres (as a rule, do not extend beyond the limits of one lobe).

2. Subtentorial:
    - in the cerebellum
    - pons.

Clinical manifestations of intracerebral hemorrhage

Determined by the amount of hemorrhage, degree and prevalence perifocal ischemia, severity of cerebral edema

Intracerebral haemorrhage

Syndrome	Clinical manifestations
Cerebral palsy	A sharp headache, nausea, vomiting, there may be epileptic attacks, a violation of consciousness (from stunning to coma)
Vegetative disorders	Skin covers are crimson-red, covered with sweat, breathing is hoarse, the pulse is strained, blood pressure is increased, hyperthermia
Lobarnoe hemorrhage, hemorrhage in the basal ganglia and internal capsule	Contralateral hemiplegia, hemianesthesia, hemianopsia, paresis of mimic muscles and language in the central type, aphasia (defeat of the dominant hemisphere), or violation of the body scheme, autopagnosia, anosognosia (defeat of the subdominant hemisphere)
Hemorrhage in the thalamus	Contralateral hemianesthesia, hemiataxia, hemianopsia, m. transient hemiparesis, amnesia, drowsiness, apathy
Hemorrhage in the cerebellum	Severe dizziness, miosis, nystagmus, repeated vomiting, severe pain in the neck and neck, hypotension or atony of the muscles, ataxia, rapid increase of intracranial hypertension
Hemorrhage in the trunk of the brain	Rapid development of deep coma, tetraplegia, decerebral rigidity, miosis (hearth in the bridge), respiratory and cardiovascular disorders. With a small size of the focus in the bridge cover, consciousness can be preserved, alternating syndromes Violation of muscle tone - dissociation along the axis, extensor pathological stop reflexes, appearance of the same type of act
Hemorrhage in the upper part of the brain stem (diencephalic and mesencephalic structures)	Defeat of the hypothalamus: tachy-, bradycardia, AH Defeat 3 pairs of CMN: pupillary reaction to light is weak or absent, divergent strabismus, paresis of the eye upward

Hemorrhage in the middle section of the brain stem (bridge)	Defeat of V-VIII pairs of CMN: suppression or complete extinction of corneal reflexes, convergent strabismus, Hertvig-Magendie symptom, prolapse of horizontal and vertical oculocephalic reflexes
Hemorrhage in the lower parts of the brainstem (bulbar departments)	Defeat of the medulla oblongata: bulbar disorders (in the patient with the intubation tube - no response to it and cough reflex), there may be bradypnoea, bradycardia, arterial hypotension

Clinical manifestations of subarachnoid hemorrhage (SAH)

There are subarachnoid, subarachnoid-parenchymal, subarachnoid-ventricular, subarachnoidal-parenchymal-ventricular CAA species.

Main clinical syndromes of subarachnoid hemorrhage

Syndrome	Clinical manifestations
Cerebral palsy	Acute development of intense headache, nausea, vomiting, there may be epileptic seizures Violation of consciousness (from stunning to coma) Psychomotor agitation
Meningeal	One of the main early symptoms in the clinical picture is photophobia, the zygomatic symptom of Bekhte-rova, then the symptoms of Kernig, Brudzinsky
Vegetative disorders (as a result of irritation with the blood flow of the hypothalamic region, spasm of its arteries)	Increased blood pressure, hyperthermia, changes in heart rate (brady-, tachycardia), changes in ECG (violation of intracardiac conduction, increased load on the right heart, negative ST interval)
Focal neurological symptoms	Usually there are no, but their presence in the early stages of the disease allows us to assume an aneurysmal genesis and establish its localization

Early focal neurological syndromes after subarachnoid hemorrhage, suggesting the presence of an aneurysm and establishing its localization

Sindrom	Supposed Cause and localization of pathological education that causes focal symptoms

Hemiparesis, hemihyesthesia is possible, aphasia hemisphere), homonymous hemianopsia	Aneurysm of the middle cerebral artery, a blood clot in the subarachnoid space of the Sylvian furrow
Headache in the paraorbital area, decreased visual acuity, loss of visual fields	Aneurysm of the internal carotid artery at the mouth of the eye artery
Mental changes in the form of emotional lability, psychomotor excitation, decreased intelligence, confabulation amnestic syndrome, possible lower paraparesis, akinetic mutism, electrolyte disturbances diabetes insipidus	Aneurysm of the anterior connective arteries
The defeat of the III pair of CMN (ptosis, mydriasis, strabismus)	Aneurysm of the internal carotid artery at the point of retreat of the posterior connective artery, rarely - the main, upper cerebellar artery or the mouth of the upper choroid artery
Defeat of the VI pair of CMN (more often bilateral)	Increase in CSF pressure
Cerebellar ataxia, Wallenberg's syndrome Zakharchenko	Stratification of the vertebral artery
One or two-way lesion III couples CHMN, symptom Parino, vertical, rotator nystagmus, ophthalmoplegia	Aneurysm of the upper segment of the main artery
Dysphagia, dysarthria, language hemiatrophy, disturbance of vibrational, temperature, pain sensitivity, dysesthesia in the legs. With a massive hemorrhage - a coma with respiratory failure	Aneurysm of the lower part of the main arteries

The development of focal neurologic symptoms at the 2-3rd week of the disease is associated, as a rule, with secondary ischemia due to vascular spasm, while the clinical picture is determined by the pool of the spasmodic artery, the degree of its narrowing and the features of the collateral circulation.

Clinical signs of secondary ischemia depending on the spasmodic artery
The defeat of the common trunk of the middle cerebral artery
Contralateral hemiparesis, hemiipesthesia, homonymous hemianopia. Turn the gaze and the head towards the focus of the cerebral infarction. Total aphasia (dominant hemisphere). Contralateral autotopagnosia, anosognosia (non-dominant hemisphere).
Single perforating branches
Contralateral predominantly brachiocephalic hemiparesis, contralateral hemianesthesia. Motor aphasia Broca (dominant hemisphere). Paresis of the eye in the opposite direction (turning the eyes toward the hearth). Buccophacial apraxia, idiomotor apraxia of extremities, contralateral autopopnosion, anosognosia.
The lower part of the middle cerebral artery
Homonymous hemianopsia. Sensory aphasia Wernicke (dominant hemisphere). Contralateral anosognosia (non-dominant hemisphere). The motor disturbances are minimal, transient in nature - sensitive disturbances are uncharacteristic. Spatial hemiagnosis, disorientation in space, visual illusions (non-dominant hemisphere), disturbances in the emotional sphere (non-dominant hemisphere).
Lenticulostrial arteries (deep branches): striatocapsular infarction
Pronounced motor (sensorimotor) hemiparesis or hemiplegia, homonymous hemianopsia
Single perforating branches
Lacunar syndromes: ☐ Purely motor hemiparesis; ☐ Purely sensory syndrome; ☐ Sensory motor hemiparesis; ☐ Cataxial hemiparesis; ☐ Disorders and awkwardness in the hand.
Anterior cerebral artery
Contralateral paresis of the foot. A less pronounced paresis of the arm is possible. Hemianesthesia, mainly in the leg. Urinary incontinence. Contralateral grasping reflex, sucking reflex. Abulically akinetic syndrome, inhibition, sluggishness, aspontaneity, whisper speech, akinetic mutism. Apraxia walking. Apraxia in the extremities (syndrome of disintegration of the corpus callosum).Emotional lability, euphoria.

Clinical signs of cerebral infarction in the vertebrobasilar artery basin

The vertebral artery, its branches and the proximal section of the basilar artery
Medial syndrome of the medulla oblongata: - on the side of defeat - paralysis and atrophy of half of the tongue;   - on the opposite side - paralysis of the arm and leg, loss of tactile and proprioceptive sensitivity.
Vertebral artery or posterior inferior cerebellar, upper, middle or lower artery of the medulla oblongata
Lateral syndrome of the medulla oblongata: - on the side of defeat - pain, violation of sensitivity on half of face, ataxia, fall to the side of defeat, nystagmus, dizziness, vomiting, syndrome Horner, dysphagia, hoarseness, soft palate paralysis, loss of taste, numbness arms, half of the trunk or legs;   - on the opposite side-loss of a vote   Temperature   sensitivity
Vertebral artery (occlusion)
Syndrome of complete transverse lesion of half of the medulla oblongata (a combination of medial and lateral syndromes of the medulla oblongata)
Lateral syndrome of the variolium bridge and medulla oblongata (combination lateral syndrome of the medulla oblongata and lateral lower syndrome of the bridge of varioly)
The basilar artery (or the only vertebral artery)
Combination of various stem syndromes and symptoms of posterior cerebral artery affection.   Two-sided damage to the conductor tracks (sensitive, motor disorders, cerebellar disorders, cranial nerve damage, tetraparesis, teraplegia, paresis and paralysis of bulbar musculature.
Paramedian branches of the distal part of the basilar artery
Paramedian branches of the distal part of the basilar artery
The medial upper syndrome of the parolysis bridge: - On the side of the lesion - cerebellar ataxia, internuclear ophthalmoplegia, myoclonia of the soft palate, pharynx, vocal cords, respiratory muscles, face, oculomotor muscles;   - on the opposite side - hemiplegia, violation of tactile, vibrational, proprioceptive sensitivity.
Upper cerebellar artery
Lateral upper syndrome of the parolysis bridge: - On the side of the focus - ataxia, falling towards the lesion, dizziness, nystagmus, vomiting, gaze toward the focus, strabismus, ptosis, myosis, anhidrosis (Horner's syndrome), tremor of rest;   - on the opposite side - violation of pain, temperature, tactile, Vibration and proprioceptive sensitivity, predominantly in the arm.
Paramedian branches of the middle part of the basilar artery
The medial medulla bridge syndrome:

- On the side of the focus - ataxia, abasia; - On the opposite side - hemiplegia, violation of tactile and proprioceptive sensitivity.
Short envelopes of the artery
Lateral median syndrome of the parolysis bridge: -On the side of the focus - ataxia, paralysis of the masticatory muscles, impaired sensitivity on half of the face; - on the opposite side - violation of pain and temperature sensitivity in the limbs and trunk.
Paramedic branches of the proximal part of the basilar artery
The medial lower syndrome of the parolysis bridge: - on the side of the focus - paresis of the eye towards the focus, nystagmus, ataxia, abasia, diplopia when looking away; - On the opposite side - hemiplegia, a violation of tactile and proprioceptive sensitivity.
Anterior lower cerebellar artery
Lateral lower syndrome of the parolysis bridge: - on the side of the focus - horizontal and vertical nystagmus, dizziness, nausea, vomiting, paralysis of mimic muscles, paresis of the eye toward the hearth, deafness, noise in the ears, ataxia, impaired sensation on the face; - on the opposite side - violation of pain and temperature sensitivity on half of the body.

Clinical signs of cerebral infarction in the basin of the posterior cerebral artery

The affected pool arteries	Clinical manifestations
Precomcommunications part (proximal connection of the compound with a backplane artery) leaving it perforating arteries	Thalamic syndromes (loss of all kinds of sensitivity, pain and dysesthesia, hemianopsia, hand spasm, mild hemiparesis), choreoathetosis, intentional tremor when the posterior ventral nuclei of the thalamusas are involved with the involvement of the subtalamic nucleus and its afferent pathways. Claude's syndrome with a lesion of the dentatotalamic pathway and the region of the exit of the oculomotor nerve: on the side of the lesion paresis of the oculomotor nerve;

	on the opposite - cerebellar ataxia. Weber's syndrome (with the defeat of the oculomotor nerve and the brain stem): on the side of the lesion paresis of the oculomotor nerve; on the opposite side - hemiplegia. Contralateral hemiplegia in the defeat of the brain stem. Paresis and paralysis of vertical eye movements, strabismus, sluggish response of pupils to light, light miosis, ptosis in the defeat of supranuclear fibers to the oculomotor nerve, Kahal's intermediate nucleus, nucleus Darksevic. Contralateral rhythmic tremor, postural tremor with ataxia, rhythmic postural tremor (dendorubralny tremor) in the lesion of the dentatalamic pathway.
Post-communication part (distal to the place connection with the backplane artery)	Homonymous hemianopsia, bilateral hemiapia, cortical blindness, awareness or negation possible blindness, apraxia of eye movements (with bilateral napolnoporazhenii occipital lobes). Memory impairments, orientation in space, simultaneous agnosia, ignoring half the field of view. Uncertain visual hallucinations, peduncular hallucinosis, metamorphosis, impaired perception of distance, distortion of contours of objects. Complex hallucinations.

Differential diagnostics
etiopathogenetic subtypes of cerebral infarction

Atherothrombotic (cerebral macroangiopathy of the TOAST classification). Occurs when the blood flow decreases or ceases on extracranial or large intracranial arteries due to atherosclerosis, atherothrombosis by constriction or complete occlusion of the protruding vessel. Risk factors: arterial hypertension, diabetes, smoking, hyperlipidemia.	Stupeneobraznoe increase in symptoms for several hours or days, often started at night. Clinical manifestations may include impairment of the functions of the cerebral cortex (aphasia, a syndrome of ignoring the opposite half of the space, limited motor deficiency), a brain stem or cerebellum. With CT and MRI, there is a cortical or subcortical hemispheric, cerebellar or stem focus, whose diameter usually exceeds 1.5 cm. In the anamnesis, indications of previous TIAs in the same vascular basin. The noise over the carotid artery or a decrease in its pulsation. According to ultrasound, MR angiography or contrast angiography on the side of IMstenosis> 50.0% of a large cerebral vessel (or its cortical branch) or an atherosclerotic plaque with an uneven surface and a parietal thrombus. The diagnosis of a stroke caused by atherosclerosis of a large artery can not be established if the ultrasound duplex examination or angiography do not show any changes or reveal minimal changes in blood vessels.
Embolic (cardioembolic). It occurs when the bladder is broken by the pathology of the chambers of the heart with the violation of wall movements, blood stagnation and hypercoagulability (ciliary arrhythmia, myocardial infarction, cardiomyopathy, myxoma, etc.), heart valves (infective endocarditis, artificial valves heart, valvular heart disease	Characterized by a sudden onset, often in the daytime against a background of physical or emotional stress. In the opening may be a violation of consciousness, an epileptic attack. The neurological deficit is most pronounced in the debut of the disease. MI is often localized in the cortical (cortical-subcortical) zonovascularization of the middle or anterior cerebral artery. Partial

and others), paradoxical cardial embolism (with defects of partitions). In addition to thrombi, the embolic substrate can be tumorous particles, bacterial and non-bacterial vegetation, myxomatous fragments, cholesterol crystals, etc.	infarcts are characteristic: isolated aphasia, hemiparesis with predominance in the arm, brachiocephalic paresis. Often there is a hemorrhagic component (according to CT or MRI). The diagnosis of cardioembolic stroke confirms the signs previous TIA or stroke in more than one vascular pool or systemic embolism.
Hemodynamic stroke. Occurs in connection with the development global hypoperfusion of the brain with a sharp decrease in blood pressure, volume circulating blood and lack accuracy of cerebral autoregulation (shock states, after surgical complications, bleeding, hypovolemia, heart failure, severe arrhythmia, orthostatic hypotension in diabetic disautonomy or inadequate antihypertensive therapy).	The diagnosis is confirmed by: anamnestic indication of a possible sharp drop in blood pressure, presence of pathology of the pre- or cerebral arteries, especially multiple and bilateral, anomalies of the cerebral vascular system (separation Willis circle, arterial hypoplasia), hemodynamically significant stenosis of the BSA with marked decrease in velocity and reserve of blood flow in all arterial basins. Given CT and MRI IM is localized in cortical or subcortical watershed zones (zones of blood supply) temporomandibular region or in the region of the convectional surface of pre- and postcentral gyri, may specular cerebral infarctions. The size of the infarct varies from small to large. The onset of a sudden with a pre-fainting or fainting condition, nausea, a sharp decrease in visual acuity and hearing, clarity of consciousness, expressed pallor of the skin. The patient's condition worsens when sitting and standing. The vegetative orthostatic is sharp or moderately positive tests. For clinical manifestations, various visual disturbances are characteristic.
Lacunar stroke (cerebral microangiopathy according to TOAST classification). Occurs in the occlusion	Debut disease: rapid development of mild or moderate neurological deficit, but there may be a gradual increase in the

of small penetrating arteries due to arteriolopathy in hypertension, diabetes mellitus, microemboli from extra cranial arteries and heart in the deep sections of the parenchyma Brain.Factors of risk: arterial hypertension, diabetes, alcoholism, chronic renal insufficiency, obstructive pulmonary diseases, constant arrhythmia, hemodynamically significant stenosis of the BCA, antiphospholipid syndrome, cerebral vasculitis and etc.	asymptomatics from a few hours to a day. May be preceded by stereotyped TIAs in the basin of small vessels. Clinic: absence of cerebral manifestations, violations of higher cortical functions. Flow by the type of small stroke. The development of lacunar syndromes: purely sensory, purely motorized hemiparesis, sensorimotor lacunar syndrome, "atactic hemiparesis" syndrome, "dysarthria and awkward brush" syndrome. According to CT, MRI - localization of the focus in white matter of the large hemispheres, subcortical ganglia, inner capsule, radiant crown, seminal shaft, bridge and trunk. The diameter of the focus of infarction is no more than 20 mm. The formulation of the diagnosis "lacunar infarction" is correct only in case of its verification using neuroimaging methods.
IM by type of hemorheological micro-occlusion develops when change of rheological properties blood leading to occlusion microcirculatory path.	The leading role of violations is characteristic rheological properties of blood and changes in the thrombocyte endothelial link of hemostasis. The main criteria for its diagnosis: the minimum severity of vascular disease (atherosclerosis, hypertension, vasculitis, vasculopathy), the presence of severe hemorheological disorders with platelet hyperactivation against the background of depletion of the antiaggregational link of endothelial hemostasis, but with a normal balance between plasma markers of hemostatic activation, fibrinolysis function and fibrinolytic potential of the vascular endothelium; expressed dissociation

	between the clinical picture (moderate neurological deficit, small size of the focus) and significant changes in blood; relative high-quality flow with rapid regression of neurological symptoms ("minor stroke"); absence of cerebral symptomatology.

Examination of patient in BIC or neurological department with the character of cerebral stroke confirmed at the admission department

Research	Ischemic stroke	Hemorrhagic stroke
Hemocoagulation	In the acute period is characteristic: - reduction of bleeding time and blood coagulation, increased fibrinogen, prothrombin, increased plasma tolerance to heparin, change in APTT (activated partial thromboplasty time); - increased adhesion and aggregation of platelets; - Reduced elasticity of erythrocyte membranes. Possible development of the syndrome of ICE with hypocoagulation, a decrease in the number of platelets, fibrinogen and prothrombin index.	In the acute period is more typical: - increased fibrinolytic activity; - with thromboelastroscopy, the onset of coagulation is delayed (2-2,5 times R is prolonged), and the coagulation time K (from the beginning of coagulation to the moment of formation of a dense clot) is decreased, the angle уменьшается decreases (lack of elasticity convolution).
Echocardiography	Signs of the pathology of the myocardium, heart defects, the presence of thrombi or myxoma in the cavities and valves of the medium.	Dilation of the heart cavities, hypertrophy of the walls of the heart.
EEG	Nonspecific for the nature of the stroke. Reflects the presence of cerebral disorders, interhemispheric asymmetry, focal changes and the development of secondary stem syndrome.	

Oculoplethysmogr aphy, ultrasound of the main arteries of the head, duplex scanning, transcranial dopplerography	There are atherosclerotic plaques and hemodynamically significant stenosis of the arteries, a decrease in the rate and a change in the direction of the blood flow along the extra- and intracranial vessels.	Identify the presence of pathology of malformations
Angiography and subtraction angiography	Supports the presence of the pathology of cerebral vessels before the planned neurosurgical intervention.	
MRI	It allows to obtain the image of the necrosis zone (infarction), to reveal the signs of perifocal edema and the displacement of the liquorodynamic pathways. In the anti-graphic mode, the image of the vessels is non-invasive.	It allows you to get images of hemorrhage and hematomas, signs of brain edema, getting into liquorodynamic pathways and their displacement.

Scale of Injuries to the National Health InstitutionNJHSS
(National Institutes of Health Stroke Scaie, Brott T., Adams H.P., 1989)

1. Level of consciousness
0 - in the mind, actively reacts.
1 - somnolence, but you can wake up with minimal irritation, perform a command, answer questions.
2 - sopor, repeated stimulation is required to maintain activity or
It is inhibited and a strong and painful stimulation is required to produce non-stereotyped movements.
3 - coma, reacts only to reflex actions or does not respond to irritants.

2. Level of consciousness: answers to questions.
Ask the patient what month and age is now. Write the first answer. If aphasia or sopor score 2. If the endotracheal tube, trauma, severe dysarthria, the language barrier – 1.
0- is the correct answer to both questions.
1 - the correct answer to one question.
2- The correct answers are not given.

3. Level of consciousness: the execution of commands.
The patient is asked to open and close his eyes, squeeze and unclench the non-paralyzed arm. Only the first attempt is counted.
    0 - both commands are correctly executed.
    1 - one command is correctly executed.
    2 - no commands are executed correctly.

4. Movement of eyeballs.
Only horizontal eye movements are counted.
    0 - is the norm.
    1 - partial paralysis of the eye.
    2 - tonic eye removal or complete paralysis of the eye, not overcome, causing oculocephalic reflexes.

5. Investigation of the fields of vision.
    0 - is the norm.
    1 - partial hemianopsia.
    2 - complete hemianopsia.

6. The section of the facial musculature.
    0 is the norm.
    1 - minimal paralysis (asymmetry).
    2 - partial paralysis - complete or almost complete paralysis of the lower muscle group.
    3 - complete paralysis (absence of movements in the upper and lower muscle groups).

7. Movement in the upper limbs.
The arms are raised at an angle of 45 ° in the supine position, at an angle of 90 ° in the sitting position. If the patient does not understand the task, the doctor should place his hands in the required position himself. Points are recorded separately for the right and left limbs.
    0 - limbs held for 10 seconds.
    1 - limbs retained for less than 10 seconds.
    2-extremities do not rise or maintain the preset position, but produce some resistance to gravity.
    3 - limbs fall without resistance to gravity.
    4- no active movements.

5- it is impossible to check (limb amputated, artificial joint).

8. Movement in the lower limbs.
In the prone position, raise the paretic leg for 5 seconds at an angle of 30 °. Points are recorded separately for the right and left extremities.

0 - the legs are held for 5 seconds.

1 - the limbs are held for less than 5 seconds.

2 - the limbs do not rise or hold the raised position, but produce some resistance to gravity.

3 - limbs fall without resistance to gravity.

4 - no active movements.

5 - can not be checked (limb amputated, artificial joint).

9. Ataxia of the extremities.
Finger - nasal and heel-knee tests are conducted from two sides, ataxia is counted in the event that it is not caused by paresis.

0 is absent.

1 - in one limb.

2 - in two extremities.

10. Sensitivity.
Only the hemiti type disorder is considered.

0 - is the norm.

1 - mild or moderate disorders.

2- Significant or complete impairment of sensitivity.

11.Afasia.
The patient is asked to describe the picture, name the subject, read the sentence.

0 - no aphasia.

1- mild aphasia.

2- pronounced aphasia.

3- complete aphasia.

12. Dysarthria.
0 - normal articulation.

1 - mild or moderate dysarthria. Do not pronounce a few words.

2 - expressed dysarthria.

3 - intubated or other physical barrier.

13. Agnosia (ignoring).
0 - there is no agnosia.
1 - ignoring one sensory modality for bilateral sequential stimulation.
2 - expressed hemiagnosis or hemiagnosis is greater than in one modality.

The Hunt and Hess Scale

It is used to assess the severity of the condition of patients with subarachnoid hemorrhage

Symptoms Items	
Headaches, mild phenomena of meningism	1
Severe headaches, pronounced phenomena of meningism, paralysis of the cranial nerves, the absence of other neurological disorders	2
Somnolent state, disturbances in the mental state of the patient, mild focal symptomatology	3
Soporous state, hemiparesis, vegetative dysregulation	4
Coma	5

Scale Coma Glasgow

It is used to assess the degree of severity of a patient with stroke, dynamics during treatment.

Symptoms	Gradations	Score
Opening the eyes	Spontaneously with blinking	4
	At the command / voice	3
	On pain stimuli	2
	Absent	1
Motor response (best response in unaffected limbs)	Executing Commands	6
	Hand localizes the place of pain stimulus	5
	Distracting the hand to the pain stimulus	4
	Bending the hand to a pain stimulus	3
	Extension of the hand to the pain stimulus	2
	Absent	1
Verbal response	Norm	5

	Confused speech	4
	Inadequate words or expressions	3
	There are distinguishable sounds, but not	2
	Absent	1

Modified Rankin scale
(UK-T1AStudyGroup, 1988)

0 - No symptoms.

1 - Absence of significant disorders of vital activity, despite the presence of some symptoms of the disease; the patient is able to perform all usual daily duties.

2 - mild disability; the patient is unable to perform some of the previous duties, but copes with his own affairs without outside help.

3 - Moderate impairment of vital functions; need for some help, but walks alone.

4 – Mfrked impairment of vital activity, can not walk without help, to cope with it's physical needs without assistance.

5- gross impairment of vital activity; confined to bed, incontinence of stool and urine, the need for constant assistance of medical personnel.

6 - Death of the patient.

Algorithm provision of prehospital, inpatient, outpatient care patients with stroke

Primary signs and symptoms of stroke requiring medical attention
1. Weakness or the appearance of embarrassment in any part of the body, especially on one half of the body, including the face, arm or leg;
2. Numbness (loss of sensation) in any part of the body, especially on one half of the body;
3. Unexplained visual impairment;
4. Violation of oral speech or understanding of speech;
5. Shakiness when walking;
6. Any other transient violations of neurological functions (dizziness, impaired swallowing, memory impairment);
7. Unusually severe, suddenly developed headache;
8. A seizure or some other unexplained disorder of consciousness.

Appeal - call an ambulance

↓

The ambulance team (no more than 40 min for the urban and no more than 3 hours for the rural population)
Arrival of the ambulance team, examination of the patient, urgent transportation to a specialized department of a multidisciplinary medical institution (stroke center)

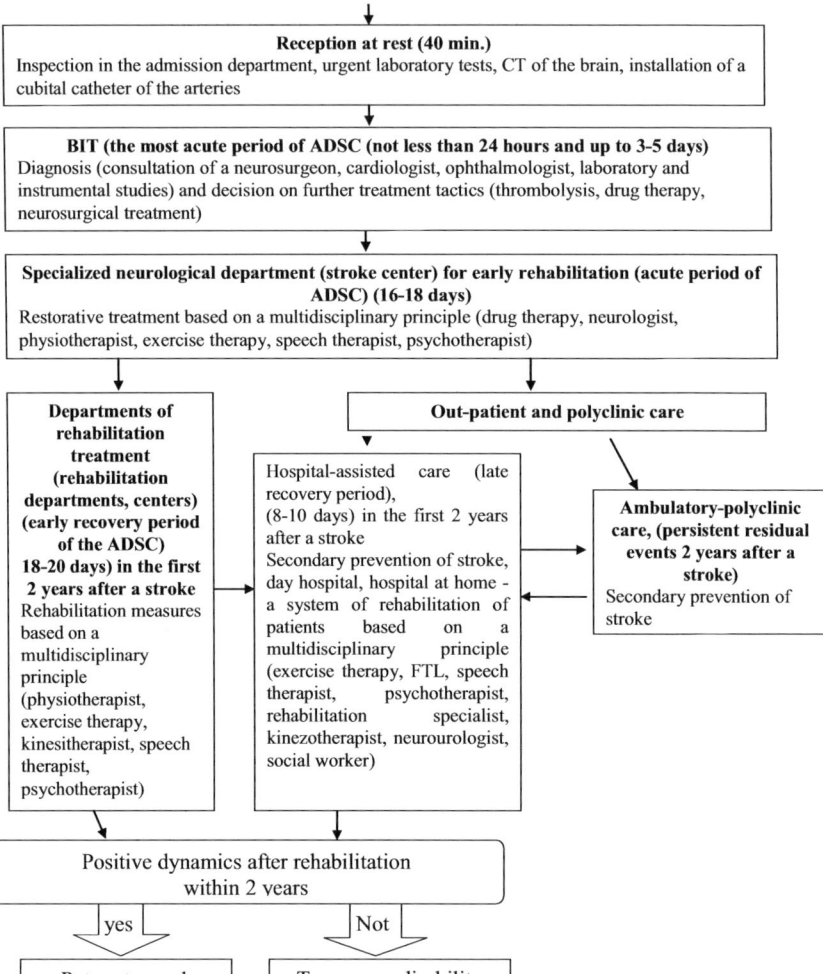

The algorithm of actions of the ambulance brigade
Prehospital stage

PHC physician, Physician PHC, patient

↓

The ambulance team (according to the clinical protocols)

↓

Functions: maintenance of vital functions and immediate delivery of the patient to the appropriate hospital.

Immediate actions of a team of emergency medical doctors upon arrival to a sick stroke should include a set of mandatory measures that are carried out immediately after a general examination of the patient (according to the protocol E-009).

- **Assessment of the adequacy of oxygenation and its correction (the inadequacy of oxygenation is indicated by:** increased frequency and arrhythmia of respiratory movements, cyanosis of visible mucous membranes and nail lodges, participation in the act of respiration of the auxiliary musculature;
swelling of the cervical veins).

↓

To normalize breathing - toilet upper respiratory tract and oropharynx.
Anxiety is oxygen therapy. Artificial ventilation of the lungs is indicated with bradypnoea (CDP <12 per min), tachypnea (CDP> 35-40 per min), increasing cyanosis.
In the presence of arterial hypertension (systolic blood pressure> 200 mmHg, diastolic blood pressure> 110 mmHg), a slow decrease in blood pressure is shown (no more than 15-20% of the baseline values for an hour, because the sharp lowering or arterial pressure below 160/110 mm Hg are dangerous by aggravation of cerebral ischemia).
For arterial hypotension (systolic blood pressure <100 mmHg), polyglucin is injected intravenously with 400.0 ml (first 50 ml of jet) or pentastarch 500 ml. With severe arterial hypotension, intravenous drip administration of 250 mg of dopamine in 250 ml of a 5% dextrose solution or isotonic sodium chloride solution is indicated at a rate of 3-6 to 10-12 drops / min.
When a susceptible syndrome occurs: use of anticonvulsants.
In case of emergency, with a persistent hiccup: the use of antiemetics.

Algorithm of actions of the doctor of reception rest
Hospital Stage

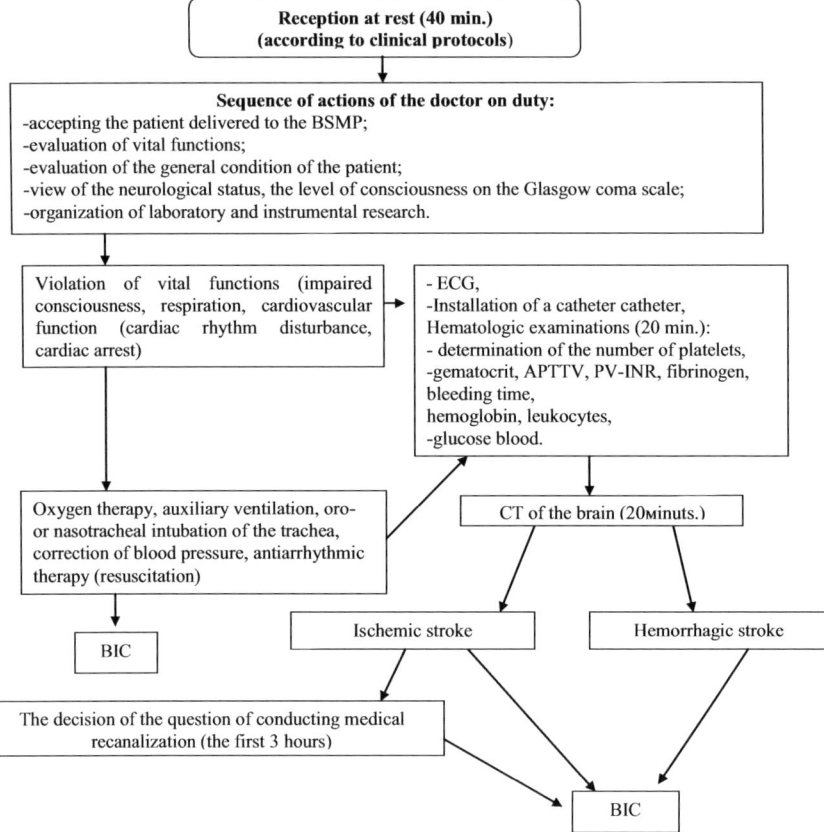

Algorithm of actions in BIT in ischemic stroke
Hospital Stage

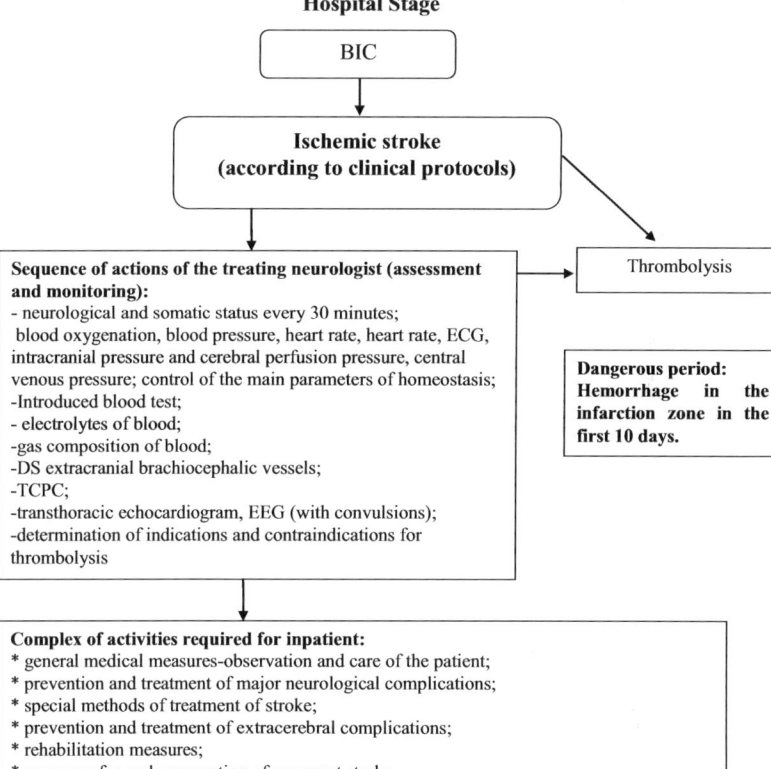

Algorithm of actions in BIC in hemorrhagic stroke (intracerebral and / or intraventricular hemorrhage)
Hospital Stage

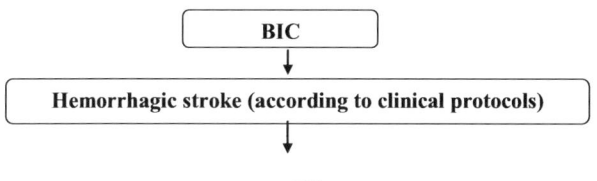

| Intracerebral and / or intraventricular hemorrhage |

Sequence of actions of the treating neurologist (assessment and monitoring):

- neurological, somatic status, level of consciousness according to Glasgow coma scale every 30 minutes;
 blood oxygenation, blood pressure, heart rate, heart rate, ECG, intracranial pressure and cerebral perfusion pressure, central venous pressure; control of the main parameters of homeostasis;
-Introduced blood test, blood electrolytes, blood gas composition, PV, APTT, blood sugar, urinalysis; chest x-ray;
- TCDC (suspicion of vasospasm) according to indications;
-MMA, cerebral arteriography (according to indications);
-EEG (if there are convulsions);
- consultation of the ophthalmologist; -consultation of the hematologist (in the absence of causes of subarachnoid hemorrhage after arteriography, hematological tests)
- consultation of a neurosurgeon to determine the indications of a neurosurgical intervention:
Indications for neurosurgical treatment:
1. patients with severe neurological deficit with signs of involvement in the pathological process of the brainstem and extensive brain hemorrhage (more than 40 cm3) according to CT;
2. Patients with focal neurological deficit in combination with easily or moderately expressed signs of involvement in the pathological process of the brainstem and CT scan with data indicating a large or average hemorrhage in the brain.

Complex of activities required for inpatient:
* general medical measures-observation and care of the patient;
* prevention and treatment of major neurological complications;
* special methods of treatment of stroke;
* prevention and treatment of extracerebral complications;
* rehabilitation measures;
* measures for early prevention of recurrent stroke.

Algorithm of actions in BIC in hemorrhagic stroke (subarachnoid hemorrhage) Hospital Stage

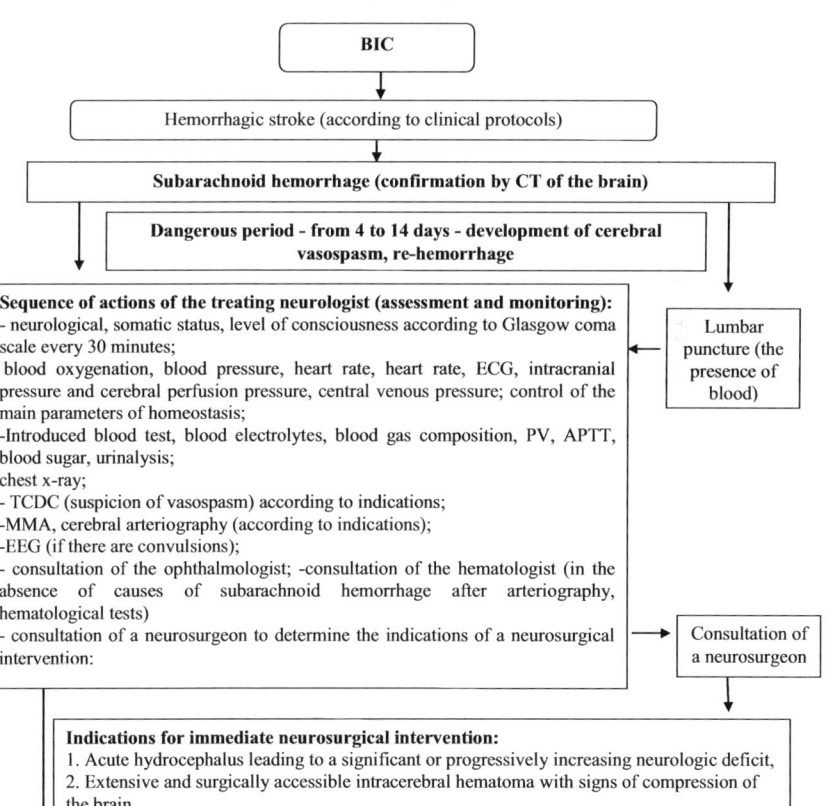

Sequence of actions of the treating neurologist (assessment and monitoring):
- neurological, somatic status, level of consciousness according to Glasgow coma scale every 30 minutes;
blood oxygenation, blood pressure, heart rate, heart rate, ECG, intracranial pressure and cerebral perfusion pressure, central venous pressure; control of the main parameters of homeostasis;
-Introduced blood test, blood electrolytes, blood gas composition, PV, APTT, blood sugar, urinalysis;
chest x-ray;
- TCDC (suspicion of vasospasm) according to indications;
-MMA, cerebral arteriography (according to indications);
-EEG (if there are convulsions);
- consultation of the ophthalmologist; -consultation of the hematologist (in the absence of causes of subarachnoid hemorrhage after arteriography, hematological tests)
- consultation of a neurosurgeon to determine the indications of a neurosurgical intervention:

Indications for immediate neurosurgical intervention:
1. Acute hydrocephalus leading to a significant or progressively increasing neurologic deficit,
2. Extensive and surgically accessible intracerebral hematoma with signs of compression of the brain,
3. Repeated hemorrhage from a previously surgically untreated (not treated) aneurysm or arteriovenous malformation, after which a complete or partial restoration of the neurological deficit is observed.

Complex of activities required for inpatient:
* general medical measures-observation and care of the patient;
* prevention and treatment of major neurological complications;
* special methods of treatment of stroke;
* prevention and treatment of extracerebral complications;
* rehabilitation measures;
* measures for early prevention of recurrent stroke.

Algorithm of the specialized neurological department of the local stroke center for early rehabilitation

---

Specialized neurological department of the local stroke center for early rehabilitation (acute ADSC period) (16-18 days) (according to clinical protocols)

↓

The sequence of actions of the treating neurologist:
- receiving a patient in the acute period of ADSC
- examination of the neurological and somatic status;
  - general and biochemical analyzes according to indications;
- electrolytes of blood according to indications;
- ECG;
- Instrumental and electrophysiological methods of examination according to indications;
- repeated consultations of experts on indications (the cardiologist, the therapist, the oculist, the vascular neurosurgeon, the urologist)

↓

The complex of measures is restorative treatment based on a multidisciplinary principle:

* rehabilitation measures (physical therapist, exercise therapy, speech therapist, psychotherapist);
* general medical measures-observation and care of the patient;
* prevention and treatment of major neurological complications;
* special methods of treatment of stroke (drug therapy - vasoactive, neuroprotective, hypotensive, anticonvulsant, hypoglycemic, hypolipidemic drugs (injectable and tableted));* prevention and treatment of extracerebral complications;
* measures to prevent recurrent stroke.

Algorithm of actions of the department of rehabilitation treatment (rehabilitation departments, centers)

Departments of rehabilitation treatment (rehabilitation departments, centers) (early recovery period of the ADSC) (18-20 days) in the first 2 years after the ADSC (according to clinical protocols)

↓

The sequence of actions of the treating neurologist:
- patient's admission in the early recovery period of ADSC
- examination of the neurological and somatic status;
  - general and biochemical analyzes according to indications;
- electrolytes of blood according to indications;
- ECG;
- Instrumental and electrophysiological methods of examination according to indications;
- consultations of experts on indications.

↓

The complex of measures is restorative treatment based on a multidisciplinary principle:

* rehabilitation measures (physiotherapist, exercise therapy, kinesotherapist, rehabilitologist, speech therapist, psychotherapist);
* general medical measures-observation and care of the patient;
* prevention and treatment of major neurological complications;
* drug therapy - vasoactive, neuroprotective, hypotensive, anticonvulsant, hypoglycemic, hypolipidemic drugs (injectable and tableted according to indications));
* prevention and treatment of extracerebral complications;
* measures to prevent recurrent stroke.

Algorithm of actions of outpatient care The complex of measures is restorative treatment based on a multidisciplinary principle:

```
┌─────────────────────────────────────┐
│   Out-patient and polyclinic care   │
│   (according to clinical protocols) │
└─────────────────────────────────────┘
```

Hospital-assisted care (late recovery period), (8-10 days) in the first 2 years each year after a stroke of the initial period), (8-10 days) in the first 2 years each year after a stroke

Ambulatory-polyclinic care, (persistent residual events 2 years after a stroke)

Functions of the neurologist:
- admission of the patient in the late recovery period of the ADSC
- referral to a day hospital and a hospital at home;
- examination of the neurological and somatic status;
- laboratory, instrumental and electrophysiological research methods according to indications;
- secondary prevention of stroke;
- consultations of experts on indications;
- direction and registration at the Ministry of Energy

Functions of the neurologist:
- observation and examination of patients with residual phenomena of ADSC;

The complex of measures is restorative treatment based on a multidisciplinary principle:

* rehabilitation measures (physical therapist, exercise therapy, kinesotherapist, rehabilitation specialist, speech therapist, psychotherapist, social worker);
* drug therapy - vasoactive, neuroprotective, hypotensive, anticonvulsant, hypoglycemic, hypolipidemic drugs (injectable and tabletted according to indications));

Algorithm for managing a patient with a cerebral infarction
- Raising the head end of the bed at an angle of 30^0.
- When hemiplegia - elastic stocking on the paralyzed lower limb,
- Ensuring the patency of the upper respiratory tract, feeding oxygen through a nasal probe at a rate of 2-4 l / min,
- Transfer to mechanical ventilation with tachypnea (BH> 40 / min), PaO2 <60 mmHg.
- Maintenance of normothermia,
- Analgesics:
  metamizole 50% rr 2 ml IM or IV, tramadol 1-2 ml (50-100 mg) IM (MSD -400 mg).
- At a blood glucose concentration of 10 mmol / L and above, a detailed insulin administration with regard to the level of glycemia, regardless of the presence or absence of diabetes mellitus in the anamnesis.
- Installation of a urinary catheter, a gastric probe to patients in a state of stunning-coma.
- In the first day of the stroke, correction of blood pressure is performed with SBP> 220 mmHg, DBP> 105 mmHg. (with concomitant heart failure, stratified aneurysm of the aorta, acute myocardial infarction, acute renal failure, indications for thrombolysis or intravenous administration of heparin, correction of blood pressure at lower digits). BP is reduced by 10-15% of the baseline within 24 hours. Drugs that do not adversely affect autoregulation of the cerebral blood flow and are easily titrated are preferred: captopril 12.5 mg orally if the blood pressure decreases by 30% , repeated reception of 12,5 mg in 3 hours if the arterial pressure has not changed or has raised - 25 mg inside; Enalapril 10-20 mg / day in 2 divided doses. With DBP> 140 mm Hg. (double measurement with an interval of 5 minutes) - nitroglycerin 20-400 μg / min IV in under the control of blood pressure. Maintaining blood pressure at the achieved level, preventing the rise and fall of blood pressure. Enalapril 10-20 mg / day in 2 doses, propranolol 20-40 mg / day in 2-3 doses, metoprolol 0.1-0.2 g / day in 2-3 doses.
- Arterial hypotension (SBP below 110 mmHg):
  Volume substitution therapy - hydroxyethyl starch 6% or 10% rp 250-500 ml / day, 10% rr dextran / sodium chloride 250-400 ml / day (counter-indications: acute myocardial infarction, arrhythmias). In the absence of the effect: dopamine 0.5% solution of 10 ml (50 mg) in 250 ml of 0.9% sodium chloride solution in / in the drip 2-5 μg / kg / min. Depending on the hemodynamic effect (blood pressure, heart rate), the rate of administration is changed to 20 μg / kg / min.
- Coagulopathy (PI <60%, APTT> 35 seconds): fresh-frozen plasma 400-1000 ml / day in / drip (before the normalization of the coagulogram).
  Correction of paroxysms of heart rhythm disturbance.

Correction of hypercholesterolemia, dyslipidemia.

- Cerebral edema, increased intracranial pressure, not decreasing on the background of sedation and / or analgesia, sodium plasma level less than 150 mmol / l (control of electrolytes at least 2 times / day): mannitol 15% r-1 g / kg in within min in combination with iv administration of 40 mg furosemide, then, taking into account the clinical manifestations and the level of osmolarity of the plasma (no more than 295 mmol / kg), the introduction of 0.25 g / kg every 4-5 hours continues.

Osmodiuretics are contraindicated in renal failure, pulmonary edema, decompensated heart failure. Hypoalbuminemia: 5% or 10% solution of albumin iv in 200 ml 1 -2 times / day.

- Antibacterial agents for suspected infection of the respiratory or urinary tracts as agreed with the physician by the therapist.

- Convulsive syndrome, diazepam 0.5% r-2ml (10 mg) iv or m / m (MSD - 60 mg); carbamazepine 200 mg 1-2 times / day with a dose increase up to 800-1200 mg / day (MSD 1600 mg / day); clonazepam 0.5-2 mg 1-4 times / day, preparations of valproic acid 300 mg 2 times / day with a dose increase up to 900-1500 mg / day (MSD 3000 mg).

- Epileptic status: diazepam iv 0.5% r-2-6 ml - 10-30 mg (0.15-0.4 mg / kg) at a rate of 2.5 mg / min, if necessary, repeatedly through 10-20 min. Perhaps iv drip diazepam in a dose of 0.1-0.2 mg / kg / h; thiopental sodium IV, | bolusno 100-250 mg per 20 seconds, then 50 mg bolus every 2-3 minutes until the seizure, then a constant infusion of 3-5 mg / kg / hour (sodium thiopental is used to arrest epileptic status only if there is a possibility of transferring the patient to IVL); phenobarbital 2-10 mg / kg / day, phenytoin 15-20 mg / kg / day, carbamazepine 800-1200 mg / day in crushed form through the nasogastric tube.

- Psychomotor agitation: diazepam 0.5% rr 2 ml (10 mg) iv or in / m; Chlorprothiksen 15-50 mg / day orally in 2-3 doses or 1 -2 ml 2.5% of r-ra w / m;

- Vomiting: metoclopramide 0.5% rr 2 ml IM or iv -1 -3 times / day;

- Vestibular syndrome: betahistine 16 mg 3 times / day or 24 mg 2 times / day inside.

- Antidepressants: amitriptyline 25 mg orally 2-3 times / day; fluoxetine 20-60 mg / day in 1-2 oral administration; paroxetine 20 mg orally 1 time / day.

- With increasing hemoglobin, erythrocytosis: 10% rr dextran / sodium chloride 250-400 ml / day IV drip for 30-60 min. 1-2 times / day 5-7 days (before the decrease of hematocrit by 10-15% or reaching the level of hematocrit 33-35%).

- Antiplatelets: acetylsalicylic acid inside the first day of the stroke 325 mg, then at a dose of 1 mg / kg / day (50-150 mg / day).

- Anticoagulants:

indications for prescribing (including APTT, platelet count, neuroimaging data): an embolic stroke with a high risk of repeated embolization; extra- and intracranial stenoses with a clinic of repeated TIA; progressive stroke; coagulopathy; DIC-syndrome; Dissection of extracranial arteries with clinical symptoms;

contraindications to the appointment: coma 3 items; extensive cerebral infarction (more than 50% of the basin of the middle cerebral artery); internal bleeding; high level of blood pressure (200/100 mm Hg and above); epileptic seizures; severe damage to the kidneys, liver; craniocerebral trauma.

Heparin in the first day of 5-10 thousand units in / in the air, then infusion 5-10 thousand units at a rate of 12-15 ED / kg / h or 2.5-5 thousand ED 4 times per day subcutaneously in perepupochnuyu cellulose. Then, 2.5-5 thousand units 4 times a day, subcutaneously in perivapochnaya fiber, 5-7 days with a gradual decrease in dose and subsequent transfer to indirect anticoagulants or antiaggregants. Prevention of thromboembolic complications: low molecular weight heparins - enoxaparin 1 mg / kg p / to 2 times / day 3-8 days, supraparin 0.1 ml / 10 kg p / to 6 days; Dalteparin - 120 IU / kg 2 times / day p / k.

Anticoagulants of indirect action appoint 3-4 days before cancellation

heparin in cardioembolic stroke, aneurysm of the main artery, arterial dissection, antiphospholipid syndrome: fenindion 30-60 mg / day in 2-3 oral doses; warfarin 2.5-5 mg / day inside. The target level of MHO is 2.0-3.0; at the age of 70-75 years - 1,4-1,7; in the presence of artificial heart valves - 2.5-3.5 (a combination with acetylsalicylic acid 50 mg / day is possible). Control MHO first 5-7 days daily or every other day, then 1-2 times a week. After stabilizing MHO at the target level - 1 time in 2-3 weeks. Xanthinal nicotinate 15% r-2 ml w / m 1-3 times / day, if necessary, activation of fibrinolysis.

- Neuroprotectors:

Magnesium sulfate 25% solution 10-20 ml iv, droplet, glycine sublingually up to 1 g / day in 3 doses, emoksipin 3% r 10-15 ml iv, choline alfoscerate (cerebro, gliatilin) 1000 mg / day intravenously, then 1200 mg / day in 3 doses, hydrolyzed peptides of the brain 10-20 ml iv, semax 12-18 mg / day intranasal, actovegin 400-800 mg / day (10-20 ml) IV, cerebrolysin 30-50ml IV, citicoline 500-1000 mg iv 1-2 times / day. At the end of the acute period (up to 3 weeks), the course of restorative treatment:

- Continue reception of anticoagulants of indirect action (fenindion, warfarin) under the control of MHO (PTI) or antiplatelet drugs.

- Neuroprotectors:

Piracetam 20% r-10 ml iv or 5 ml w / m, then inside 2.4-3.6 g / day; glycine 100 mg for 1-2 tablets. sublingual 3-5, once / day; emoksipin 3% rr 5 ml IM; vinpocetine 10 mg (4 ml) iv drip 1 -2 times / day, then 10 mg 3 times / day inside; pentoxifylline 2% r-5-10 ml iv, choline alfoscerate (cerebro, gliatilin) 1000 mg / day iv, then 1200 mg / day in 3 divided doses, semax 12-18 mg / day intranasal, actovegin 400 -800 mg / day (10-20 ml) IV, citicoline 500-1000 mg IV.

- Vestibular Syndrome:
betahistine 16 mg 3 times / day or 24 mg 2 times / day inside.
- With spasticity, muscle relaxants of central action:
baclofen 5 mg 2-3 times / day, the dose can be gradually increased to 60-70 mg / day;
Tolperisone 50-150 mg times a day.
Anticholinesterase drugs:
ipidakrin 1,5% r-2 ml IM or 20 mg 2-3 times / day inside.

Algorithm for managing a patient with subarachnoid hemorrhage
- Safety mode.
- Ensuring the patency of the upper respiratory tract, oxygen supply through the nasal probe at a rate of 2-4 l / min. Transfer to mechanical ventilation pritachipnoe (BH> 40 / min), PaO2 <60 mmHg.
- Raising the head end of the bed at an angle of 30 °.
- Analgesia and sedation during all manipulations.
- Maintenance of normothermia.
- Analgesics: metamizole 50% rr 2 ml IM or IV, tramadol 1-2 ml (50-100 mg) IM (MOD-I 400 mg).
- Correction of blood glucose concentration: 10 mmol / l and above - fractional insulin administration taking into account the level of glycemia, regardless of the presence or absence of diabetes mellitus in the anamnesis.
- Installation of a urinary catheter, a gastric probe to patients who are in a state of stunning - coma.
- Correction of blood pressure: the recommended level of SBP before clipping aneurysm 120-150 mm Hg. With an increase in blood pressure and for the prevention of angiospasm, nimodipine is 60 mg orally 4-6 times a day for 2-3 weeks (if swallowed - through a nasogastric tube). Nimodipine is contraindicated in patients with persistent arterial hypotension, tachy ¬ cardia, marked edema of the brain, aortic stenosis, decompensated heart failure. If it is possible to monitor blood pressure in the IV administration of 1 mg of nimodipine for 2 hours (15 mg / kg / h), then 2 mg for 3 hours (30 µg / kg / h) 1 time / day for 5-7 days with subsequent ingestion within 10 days. ACE inhibitors: captopril 6.25-12.5 mg, enalapril 10-20 mg. With DBP> 140 mm Hg. (based on the results of a two-fold measurement with an interval of 5 minutes): nitroglycerin 0.1%, 0.3%, 0.5% p-r, diluted 0.9% with sodium chloride to 0.005%, 0.01% p -ra, at a rate of 5-10 µg / min - 200 µg / min IV in under the control of blood pressure.
- Arterial hypotension (SBP below 110 mmHg):
volume substitution therapy - hydroxyethyl starch 6% or 10% rp 250-500 ml / day, 10% rr dextran / sodium chloride 250-400 ml / day), contraindications: acute

myocardial infarction, arrhythmias. In the absence of the effect: dopamine 0.5% solution of 10 ml (50 mg) in 250 ml of 0.9% sodium chloride solution in / in the drip 2-5 μg / kg / min. Depending on the hemodynamic effect (blood pressure, heart rate), the rate of administration is changed to 20 μg / kg / min.

- Prevention of vascular spasm and brain ischemia:

ZN therapy (hypervolemic hypertonic hemodilution) after clipping of an aneurysm with the achievement of CVP of 10-12 mm of water. stems, hematocrit 30-35%, SBP up to 200 mm Hg. Combination of colloidal and crystalloid solutions, total amount of infusion of at least 3000 ml / day.- Maintenance of normovolemia or moderate hypervolaemia under the control of venous pressure and diuresis. With CVP less than 8 cm of water: in / in the introduction of colloidal and crystalloid solutions in a ratio of 1: 1 or 1: 2, a total volume of not more than 1.5 liters / day. With CVP more than 8 cm.v.st. .: iv injection of crystalloid solutions up to 1 liter. Hydroxyethyl starch 6%, 10% rp 250-500 ml / day, 10% rr dextran / sodium chloride 250-400 ml / day. Coagulopathy (PTI <60%, APTT> 35 s):

fresh frozen plasma 400-1000 ml / day in / drip (before the normalization of the coagulogram).

- Brain edema, increased intracranial pressure, not decreasing in the background of sedation and / or analgesia, plasma sodium level less than 150 mmol / l (control of electrolytes at least 2 times / day): mannitol 15% rr 1 g / kg for 30 minutes in combination with iv administration of 40 mg furosemide. Taking into account the clinical manifestations and plasma osmolality level (no more than 295 mmol / kg) continue the introduction of 0.25 g / kg every 4-5 hours. Contraindications to the introduction of osmodiuretics: renal failure, pulmonary edema, cardiac failure. With hypoalbuminemia: 5% or 10% of the r-r albumin IV in 200 ml 1 -2 times / day. Dexamethasone 8-10 mg / m or IV, then 4 mg every 4-6 hours.

- Antibiotic therapy: if there is a suspicion of an infection of the respiratory or urinary tracts as agreed with the physician by the therapist.

- Neuroprotectants: magnesium sulfate 25% rr 10-20 ml IV drip, glycine sublingually up to 1 g / day in 3 doses, emoksipin 3% rp 10-15 ml iv, choline alfoscerate (gliatilin) 1000 mg / day IV, then 1200 mg / day in 3 divided doses, Semax 12-18 mg / day intranasally, Actovegin 400-800 mg / day (10-20 ml) IV, cortexin 10 mg IM.

- Convulsive syndrome: diazepam 0.5% solution of 2 ml (10 mg) iv or in / m (MSD - 60 mg); Carbamazepine 200 mg 1 -2 times / day with a dose increase up to 800-1200 mg / day (MSD - 1600 mg / day), i clonazepam 0.5-2 mg 1-4 times / day, preparations of valproic acid 300 mg 2 times / day with increasing the dose to 900-1500 mg / day (MSD-3000 mg).

- Epileptic status:

diazepam 0.5% rr 2-6 ml - 10-30 mg (0.15-0.4 mg / kg) IV 2.5 mg / min. The introduction can be repeated after 10-20 minutes. It is possible iv droplet injection of diazepam in a dose of 0.1-0.2 mg / kg / h), sodium thiopental in / in the air at 100-250 mg per 20 seconds, then | 50 mg bolus every 2-3 minutes until the attacks stop, then a constant infusion of 3-5 mg / kg / h (use of sodium thiopental only if there is a possibility of transferring the patient to the ventilator); phenobarbital 2-10 mg / kg / day, phenytoin 15-20 mg / kg / day, carbamazepine 800-1200 mg / day in crushed form through the nasogastric tube.

- Psychomotor agitation: diazepam 0.5% solution of 2 ml (10 mg) IV or IM; Chlorprotixen 15-50 mg / day orally in 2-3 doses or 1 -2 ml 2.5% of r-ra IM.

Vomit: metoclopramide 0.5% rp 2 ml IM or iv -1 -3 times / day.

Algorithm for conducting a patient with intracerebral hemorrhage

- Raising the head end of the bed at an angle of 30 °, with hemiplegia -

elastic stocking on the paralyzed lower limb. - Provision of patency of the upper respiratory tract, oxygen supply, a transponder probe at a rate of 2-4 l / min.

- Transfer to mechanical ventilation with tachypnea (BH> 40 / min), PaO2 <60 mmHg.

- Maintenance of normothermia.

- Analgesics: metamizole 50% rr 2 ml IM or IV, tramadol 1-2 ml (50-100 mg) IM (MSD -400 mg).

- Correction of blood glucose concentration: 10 mmol / l and above - fractional insulin administration taking into account the level of glycemia, regardless of the presence or absence of diabetes mellitus in the anamnesis.

- Installation of a urinary catheter, a gastric probe to patients in a state of stunning-coma.

- Monitoring of blood pressure: every 30 minutes the first 8 hours, then every hour during the first day: with SBP> 180 mmHg. and DBP> 105 mmHg. BP reduces no more than 20% of the initial within 1-1.5 h. (up to 160-150 / 80-85 mm Hg, average BP 120 mm Hg) with subsequent maintenance at this level.

- Cupping AG, prevention of angiospasm:

nimodipine 60 mg orally 4-6 times / day 2-3 weeks (if swallowed - through the nasogastric tube). Contraindications: persistent arterial hypotension, tachycardia, marked cerebral edema, aortic stenosis, heart failure). ACE inhibitors: captopril 6.25-12.5 mg, enalapril 10-20 mg orally.

With DBP> 140 mm Hg. (twice a measurement after 5 minutes): nitroglycerin 20-400 μg / min IV in under the control of blood pressure. With blood pressure less than 180 mm Hg. active antihypertensive therapy is not performed (with the exception of concomitant myocardial infarction, exfoliating aortic aneurysm, etc.).

- Arterial hypotension (SBP below 110 mm Hg): volume substitution therapy - hydroxyethyl starch 6% or 10% rp 250-500 ml / day, 10% rr dextran / sodium chloride 250-400 ml / day. Counter-indications: concomitant myocardial infarction, arrhythmias. In the absence of the effect: dopamine 0.5% solution of 10 ml (50 mg) in 250 ml of 0.9% sodium chloride solution in / in the drip 2-5 μg / kg / min. Depending on the hemodynamic effect (blood pressure, heart rate), the rate of administration is changed to 20 μg / kg / min.

- Brain edema, increased intracranial pressure, not decreasing on the background of sedation and / or analgesia, sodium plasma level less than 150 mmol / l (control of electrolytes at least 2 times per day): mannitol 15% r-1 g / kg in for 30 minutes in combination with iv administration of 40 mg furosemide, then taking into account the clinical manifestations and plasma osmolality level (no more than 295 mmol / kg) continue the dose of 0.25 g / kg every 4-5 hours. Contraindications to the introduction of osmodiuretics: renal failure, pulmonary edema, heart failure.

Hypoalbuminemia: 5% or 10% Sol albumin v/v in 200 ml 1-2 times / day.

- Specific pathogenetic therapy (aimed at stopping bleeding and lysis of the blood clot) has no bleeding to the brain per se, with the proviso that the maintenance of optimal blood pressure (described in basic therapy) and surgical means of hematoma evacuation are pathogenetic methods of treatment. Specific methods also include neuroprotection and reparative therapy. Coagulopathy (PTI <60%, APTT> 35 sec): fresh-frozen plasma 400-1000 ml / day in / drip (before the normalization of the coagulogram).

- Convulsive syndrome: diazepam 0.5% rr 2 ml (10 mg) iv or in / m (MSD - 60 mg), carbamazepine 200 mg 1-2 times / day with a dose increase of up to 800-1200 mg / day (MSD - 1600 mg / day), clonazepam 0.5-2 mg 1-4 times / day, preparations of valproic acid 300 mg 2 times / day with increasing the dose to 900-1500 mg / day (MSD - 3 g);

- Epileptic status:

diazepam iv / 0.5% rp 2-6 ml - 10-30 mg (0.15-0.4 mg / kg) 2.5 mg / min. If necessary, again after 10-20 minutes. It is possible iv drip diazepam in a dose of 0.1-0.2 mg / kg / h; thiopental sodium IV bolus in a dose of 100-250 mg for 20 seconds, then 50 mg bolus every 2-3 minutes until seizures stop, then a constant infusion of 3-5 mg / kg / hour (sodium thiopental for epicot cupping is used only for availability of the possibility of transferring the patient to mechanical ventilation); phenobarbital 2-10 mg / kg / day, phenytoin 15-20 mg / kg / day, carbamazepine 800-1200 mg / day in crushed form through nasogastric tube;

- Psychomotor agitation: diazepam 0.5% r-r 2 ml (10 mg) iv or in / m; Chlorprothiksen 15-50 mg / day orally in 2-3 doses or 1 -2 ml 2.5% of r-ra w / m;

- Vomiting: metoclopramide 0.5% rr 2 ml IM or IV -1 -3 times / day.

- Neuroprotectants: magnesium sulfate 25% rr 10-20 ml intravenous drip, glycine sublingually up to 1 g / day in 3 doses, emoksipin 3% rp 10-15 ml iv, choline alfoscerate (cerebro, gliatilin) 1000 mg / day IV, then 1200 mg / day in 3 divided doses, Semax 12-18 mg / day intranasally, Actovegin 400-800 mg / day (10-20 ml) IV, cerebrolysin 20-30 ml in / in.

At the end of the acute period (up to 3 weeks), the course of restorative treatment

- Neuroprotectors:

Piracetam 20% r-10 ml iv or 5 ml IM, then inside 2.4-3.6 g / day, cerebrolysin 10-20 ml w / w, glycine 100 mg for 1-2 tablets. sublingual 3-5 times a day, emoksipin 3% rp 5 ml IM, vinpocetine 10 mg (4 ml) iv drip 1 -2 times / day, then 10 mg 3 times / day inside, pentoxifylline 2% r-p 5-10 ml iv, choline alfoscerate 1000 mg / day iv, then 1200 mg / day in 3 doses, semax 12-18 mg / day intranasal, actovegin 400-800 mg / day (10- 20 ml) IV.

Systemic thrombolytic therapy with cerebral infarction

Indications for systemic thrombolytic therapy

1. Clinical diagnosis of ischemic stroke (cardioembolic, atherothrombotic, lacunar subtypes).

2. The age of 18-80 years.

3. Time not more than 3 hours from the onset of the disease to the onset of thrombolysis (time "From door to needle", door-to-needletime).

5. Lack of significant clinical improvement before the onset of thrombolysis.

Contraindications to systemic thrombolytic therapy

According to the computer tomography of the brain:

1. The presence of signs of intracranial hemorrhage.

2. Gipodensivnaya area> 1/3 basin of the middle cerebral artery with a smoothed pattern of furrows and gyri.

According to clinical data:

1 . Small neurologic deficit or significant clinical improvement before starting therapy.

2. Severe stroke (clinically - more than 25 points on the scale of NIHSS).

Z. Clinical signs of subarachnoid hemorrhage, including in the absence of data for CT / MRI.

4. A seizure in the onset of a stroke.

5. Systolic blood pressure> 185 mm Hg, diastolic blood pressure> 105 mmHg.

According to anamnesis:

1. More than 3 hours from the onset of the disease and those patients in whom the exact time of the disease is unknown (stroke developed in sleep and other situations).

2. The use of heparin in the previous 48 hours before the stroke, the values of APTT, exceeding the normal parameters.

3. Patients with a history of stroke, concomitant diabetes mellitus.

4. Known hemorrhagic diathesis.

5. Patients receiving oral anticoagulants (warfarin, etc.).

6. Recent or apparent bleeding.

7. History of the central nervous system: a tumor, an aneurysm, a condition after surgery, interventions on the brain or spinal cord.

8. Hemorrhagic retinopathy, incl. with diabetes mellitus (visual impairment may indicate a hemorrhagic retinopathy).

9. Recent (less than 10 days) postponed external massage of the heart, a condition after abortion, after puncture of the central veins.

10. Bacterial endocarditis, pericarditis, acute pancreatitis.

11. Documented gastric ulcer during the last 3 months, erosion of the esophagus.

12. Arterial aneurysms, arterio-venous malformations, suspicion of aortic dissection.

13. Severe liver disease, including liver cirrhosis, hepatic insufficiency, portal hypertension, varicose veins of the esophagus and active hepatitis.

14. Serious surgical intervention or severe trauma during the last 3 months.

15. Tumors with a high risk of bleeding.

16. Pregnancy.

According to laboratory data:

1. The number of platelets is less than 100,000 / mm3.

2. Glycemia is less than 2.8 or more than 22.5 mmol / l.

3. INR> 1.7.

Algorithm for questioning patients to identify contraindications to thrombolytic therapy

(Shamalov NA, et al.)

	yes	no
1.Age from 18 to 80 years		
Data of anamnesis of the present disease		
2. Indicate the time of onset of the disease (hh / mm)		
3. Indicate the time of onset of the disease (hh / mm)		

	yes	No
4. Did the stroke develop during sleep?		
5. The symptoms occurred more than 3 hours ago?		
6. Was there a seizure in the onset of a stroke?		
Data of anamnesis of life	yes	No
7. Has the patient ever had a stroke earlier?		
8. Have there been hospitalizations for the last 3 months:		
8.1 Have any operational вмешательства?		
8.2 Was there any injury, incl. head?		
8.3 Was the patient in intensive care? (puncture center, veins)		
8.4 Was abortion performed?		
9. Did extraction of teeth last 2 weeks?		
10. Is there any menstrual bleeding now?		
11. Is the patient pregnant now?		
12. Are there indications for peptic ulcer of the stomach and duodenum for the last 3 months?		
13. Has the patient previously transferred surgery to the brain and spinal cord?		
14. Was the diagnosis of a brain tumor, an aneurysm, an arteriovenous malformation established earlier?		
15. Does the patient suffer from renal or hepatic insufficiency?		
16. Does the patient suffer from acute pancreatitis, hepatitis, endocarditis?		
17. Has there been increased bleeding earlier? Was the patient on this issue on treatment / examination?		
18. Did the patient receive a heparin, warfarin, phenilin before the stroke?		

Any noted → Thrombolysis is contraindicated

The technique of thrombolytic therapy (TLT)
Algorithm of conducting the patient in the admission department of the hospital
The neurologist
1. Acquaintance with complaints, collection of anamnesis
2. Neurological examination (NIHSS score)
3. Identification of indications and contraindications to TLT
4. The decision to conduct TLT (after receiving the results of CT and laboratory studies)

Nurse

1. Measurement of blood pressure on both hands, heart rate, ECG recording
2. Blood sampling for laboratory tests:
* a general blood test, glucose, platelets
* coagulogram (MHO, APTT)
* blood chemistry.

The doctor of the computer tomography

1. Computer tomography of the brain.
2. Conclusion on the results of the study.
If possible, performing transcranial dopplerography.
At a primary examination of the patient by a neurologist, the presence of a relative accompanying the patient is desirable to obtain reliable information about the patient and his disease.

The algorithm of conducting the patient in the intensive care intensive care unit (intensive care unit and intensive therapy of the insulin department)

1. Inspection of a patient by a reanimatologist
2. Connection of the patient to the follow-up equipment: monitoring of blood pressure, heart rate, BH, body temperature, Sa02.
3. Introduction of alteplase (only in the peripheral vein): the recommended dose of 0.9 mg / kg of body weight (maximum dose of 90 mg) - 10% of the total dose for the patient is administered as a bolus intravenously struino for 1 min, the remaining dose is administered intravenously drip for 1 hour.

Algorithm of patient management after thrombolysis

1. Evaluation of neurological status according to the NIHSS scale:
* during TLT - every 15 minutes
* up to 24 hours - every hour.
2. Control of blood pressure:
* 2 hours from the start of TLT - every 15 minutes; "6 hours - every 30 minutes;
* Up to 24 hours - every 60 minutes.3. Control computer tomography studies are conducted:
* at the end of 1-day (in the period from 22 to 36 hours)
* On the 7th day from the onset of the stroke (in the case of clinical impairment - in the earlier periods).
Important: After TLT, glycemia control is necessary, non-intercalated veins should not be punctured, catheters and probes should not be inserted within 24 hours (if necessary, prior to starting TLT). Reception of anticoagulants and anti-agents

(aspirin, warfarin, heparin, etc.) is prohibited within 24 hours. The level of SBP should not exceed 185 mm Hg. article, DBP - 105 mm Hg. Art.

Complications of thrombolytic therapy

1. Hemorrhagic complications.
There are the following types of hemorrhage associated with TLT:
1. Surface hemorrhage (usually due to puncture or damage to the vascular vessels).
2. Internal hemorrhages in the gastrointestinal or urogenital tract, in the retroperitoneal space, the central nervous system, bleeding of the paralytic organs. Hemorrhagic transformation of the cerebral infarction can be without clinical deterioration (asymptomatic) and symptomatic (with clinical deterioration> 4 on the NIHSS scale).

Algorithm for the development of hemorrhagic complications;
1. Occurrence of meningeal syndrome during or after TLT, development and increase of cerebral symptoms, significant aggravation of focal neurologic symptoms may indicate the development of hemorrhagic transformation of cerebral infarction. It is necessary to stop the introduction of alteplase, if possible repeat the CT scan and, in case of hemorrhagic transformation, begin the introduction of fresh frozen plasmas. It is also possible to use antifibrinolytic drugs (countercranial, cyclocapron), aminocaproic acid.

2. With severe bleeding (especially from places with uncompensated vents), the introduction of alteplase should be discontinued. Introduction of freshly frozen plasma is shown. Antifibrinolytic drugs (cyclocapron), aprotinin (trasilol), gordoks, aminocaproic acid can be prescribed.

3. If there is a local hemorrhage (from the injection or gum sites), discontinuation of the TLT procedure is not required.

II. Anaphylactoid reactions, orolingual edema
up to 2%, especially when taking ACE inhibitors in history.
Algorithm of actions:
• discontinuation of thrombolytic administration
• intubation
• emergency start of measures on the protocol of medical care for anaphylactic shock
• intravenous injection of fresh frozen plasma, cryoprecipitate.

ENCEPHALOPATHY

Syndrome of progressive multifocal or diffuse brain damage, manifested by clinical neurological, neuropsychological and / or mental disorders due to chronic vascular cerebral insufficiency and / or repeated episodes of cerebrovascular disorders (dyshemia, transient ischemic attack, stroke)

ALGORITHMS OF DIAGNOSIS AND TREATMENT
DISCIRCULATORY ENCEPHALOPATHY (DE)

Variants of cerebral ischemia taking into account the leading thiopathogenetic mechanism

1. Defeat of cerebral arteries of large and medium caliber ("large arterybrain disease"), caused by atherosclerosis (anomalies in the structure and divergence of the vessels are possible).

2. The defeat of small arteries and arterioles ("small artery brain disease") due to microangiopathy - hypertonic, diabetic, amyloid, inflammatory, etc.

3. Thromboembolism of brain vessels cardiogenic (atrial fibrillation, congenital and acquired heart defects, artificial valves, infarctedocardium) and arteriogenic (aortic aneurysm, atherosclerotic plaque) of nature.

4. Hemostasiopathy, a syndrome of pathological blood thickening.

5. Hypotension cardiogenic genesis, venous dysfunction, etc.

Clinical manifestations of DE

Clinical manifestations of dyscirculatory encephalopathy, stage 1	
Complaints: - headache; - noise in the head, ears, dizziness; - Rapid fatigue, absent-mindedness; снижение памяти (особенно на именаи недавние события); difficult to concentrate, fatigue when reading, writing; - decrease in working capacity in the second half of the day.	Neurological symptoms: - asymmetry of nasolabial folds, deviation of the tongue; - reflexes of oral automatism; - asymmetry of reflexes, mild impairment of sensitivity, coordination.
	Intelligence: - mild cognitive impairment.
Summary: subjective disorders dominate, accompanied by a rough neurological symptomatology, psychological testing reveals asthenic manifestations and memory loss of mild degree. With adequate therapy, a decrease in severity or elimination of symptoms is possible.	
Clinical manifestations of dyscirculatory encephalopathy, stage 2	
Complaints: - headache;	Neurological symptoms: Syndromes are revealed:

- noise of wushars, head, dizziness; - memory loss; - change of gait; - stiffness, lack of coordination, gait, change in speech.	- a pyramid, - Stem-cerebellum, - extrapyramidal and others.
Intelligence: criticism is reduced, reappraisal of one's abilities and performance, a viscosity, changes in character and behavior, moderate cognitive impairments develop.	
Summary: The frequency and severity of memory disorders, disability, dizziness, and instability in walking are increasing. The focal asymptomatic becomes more distinct, at this stage it is possible to isolate the dominant neurological syndromes- coordinator, pyramidal, amyostatic, and others. Increased severity of cognitive impairment. These manifestations significantly reduce the professional and social adaptation of patients.	
Clinical manifestations of dyscirculatory encephalopathy, stage 3	
Morphological changes in the brain tissue are diffuse and extensive. - Patients stop complaining.	Neurological symptoms: expressed neurological disorders:
Intelligence: the changes in the psyche are increasing, often reaching the state dementia, behavior changes dramatically patient.	- pseudobulbar, - Extrapyramidal, - a pyramid, - cerebellar and other syndromes. A combination of several syndromes.
Summary: The number of complaints is decreasing. Progress in reducing criticism to its state. Objective neurological disorders are aggravated, paroxysmal conditions (falls, faints, epileptic seizures) are more often observed. This stage differs from the previous one, and the fact that the patient reveals a combination of several sufficiently pronounced syndromes, which indicates a multi-oedemuscular lesion of the brain, changes in the psyche reach a degree of dementia. Patients are disabled, social and household disadaptation is observed.	

For the diagnosis of dyscirculatory encephalopathy are necessary:

1. The presence of signs of brain damage with the formation of a complex of psychopathological (emotional-volitional, cognitive) and motor (pseudobulbar, pyramidal, amyostatic, coordinator, etc.) disorders, confirmed by clinical and instrumental studies.

2. Presence of signs of acute or chronic brain dyskirculation (vascular risk factors, systemic vascular diseases, vascular lesions, confirmed by special examination methods).

4. The presence of a causal relationship of hemodynamic disorders with the development of clinical symptoms.

Treatment of dyscirculatory encephalopathy includes:

1. Adequate therapeutic effect on the main vascular disease, which is the cause of chronic cerebral vascular insufficiency (atherosclerosis, AH, etc.)

2. Prevention of ADSC (drug and surgical).

3. Restoration of cerebral blood flow.

4. Improvement of cerebral metabolism.

The main drugs used to treat dyscirculatory encephalopathy

- emoksipin 3% rr 10-15 ml IV or 5 ml IM;
- vinpocetine (Cavinton) 10-20 mg (4-8 ml) IV, after the course of infusions 10 mg
- 3 times / day inside for a long time;
- pentoxifylline 2% rr 5-10 ml iv;
- xanthinal nicotinate 15% r-p2ml / m1-2 times / sutil0.15-0.3 g inside3 times / day;
- glycine 100 mg for 1-2 tablets. sublingual 3-5 times / day;
- choline alphoscerate (gliatilin) 1000 mg / day IV, then 1200 mg / day
- in 2 doses (800 + 400) inside for a long time;
- mexibel 5% rr 2-4 ml (100-200 mg) iv or 2 ml (100 mg) IM 1-2 times / day, then
- 125 mg 3 times / day inside;
- Semax 4-12 mg / day intranasally in 2-3 divided doses;
- Nicergoline 5-10 mg 3 times / day inside, 4 mg IV or IM;
- extract of ginkgo biloba (tanakan) 40 mg 3 times / day inside;
- citicoline 500-1000 mg IV or IM 1-2 times / day;
- deproteinized hemoderivat from the blood of calves (actovegin) 400-800 mg / day (10-20 ml) IV or 200 mg / day (5 ml) IM;
- Cerebrolysin 20ml IV 5 days a week up to 4 weeks
- Pyracetam 20% r-10 ml IV or 5 ml IM, then inside 2.4-3.6 g / day.

With vestibular syndrome:
- betahistine 16 mg 3 times / day or 24 mg 2 times / day inside.
   o In case of akinetic-rigid syndrome:
- antiparkinsonics: amantadine 50-100 mg / day 2 times / day, then 3 times / day;

- Muscle relaxants of central action: tolperisone 50-150 mg 3 times / day, up to 450 mg / day; "anticholinesterase drugs: neostigmine methyl sulfate 0.05% solution 1-2 ml / k; ipidakrin 0.5% or 1.5% solution 1 ml IM or inside 20 mg 3 times / day.
o In case of agitation, psychotic disorders, depression:
o anxiolytics: diazepam 0.5% solution (5-10 mg) IV or IM; alprazolam 0.25-1 mg 3 times / day inside, chlorprotixen 15-50 mg / day inward in 2-3 doses;- antidepressants: fluoxetine 10 mg / day inside, amitriptyline 12,5-25 mg 2-3 times / day inside, paroxetine 20 mg / day in 1 intake.
 - With epileptic seizures:
 - carbamazepine 200-400 mg / day inward, clonazepam 0.5-2 mg 1-4 times / day inward, preparations of valproic acid 300-1500 mg / day orally in 3 divided doses.
o In consultation with the therapist:
 - People with hypertension are prescribed long-term antihypertensive therapy with gradual achievement of target blood pressure levels;
 - correction of hypercholesterolemia, dyslipidemia;
 - administration of antiplatelet agents: acetylsalicylic acid 50-150 mg / day inwards, with intolerance to acetylsalicylic acid - dipyridamole 225 mg / day in 1 -3 priema inside;
 - with a high risk of vascular complications (with combined vascular pathology, several risk factors, pronounced hyperaggregation syndrome, after surgery on the vessels) - clopidogrel 75 mg / day.

Epilepsy

According to the definition of the International Antiepileptic League (IPEL) and the International Bureau of Epilepsy, epilepsy is a brain disorder characterized by a persistent predisposition to the generation of epileptic seizures, as well as neurobiological, cognitive, psychological and social disorders of this condition. The definition of epilepsy requires the appearance of at least one epileptic seizure.

Epileptic seizure is a transient occurrence of signs and / or symptoms due to abnormal excess or hypersynchronous neuronal activity in the brain.

The diagnosis of epilepsy includes 1) the establishment of an epileptic disorder, 2) the type of seizure and localization of epileptic focus (or generalized type of disorder), 3) the elucidation of the etiology of the disease, and 4) the attribution of epileptic disorders to a specific clinical form, Classification of epilepsy and epileptic syndromes. Diagnosis of epilepsy requires knowledge of the clinical and electroencephalographic picture of the variety of epileptic seizures, syndromes and forms of epilepsy.

INTERNATIONAL CLASSIFICATION OF EPILEPSIA AND EPILEPTIC SYNDROME (RECOMMENDED IN 1989 INTERNATIONAL LEAGUE AGAINST EPILEPSIA

1. EPILEPSIA AND SYNDROME WITH LOCALIZED ACCIDENTS

1.1 Idiopathic forms (the onset of seizures is associated with age):
- Benign epilepsy of children with central-temporal (Rolandic) peaks on EEG;
- Epilepsy of children with occipital paroxysms on EEG;
- Primary epilepsy of reading.

1.2. Symptomatic forms:
- Chronic pro-partial partial epilepsy of children (Kozhevnikov's syndrome);
- Syndromes with specific causes of provocation of attacks (reflex epilepsy);
- Frontal, temporal, parietal, occipital lobar epilepsy.

1.3. Cryptogenic forms (undefined forms)

2. EPILEPSIA AND SYNDROMES WITH GENERALIZED ACCIDENTS

2.1. Idiopathic (the onset of seizures is associated with age):
- Benign neonatal family convulsions;
- Benign neonatal cramps;
- Benign infantile myoclonic epilepsy;
- Epilepsy with pycnoleptic absences (pycnoplesis, absens-epilepsy of children);
- Teenage absences-epilepsy;
- Epilepsy with impulsive small attacks (adolescent myoclonic epilepsy);
- Epilepsy with generalized tonic-clonic convulsions upon awakening;
- Other forms of generalized idiopathic epilepsy;
- Epilepsy with specific provoking factors (reflex and start-epilepsy).

2.2. Cryptogenic or symptomatic forms (associated with the age of onset of seizures):
- Vest syndrome;
- Lennox-Gastaut syndrome;
- Epilepsy with myoclonic-astatic seizures;
- Epilepsy with myoclonic absences.

2.3. Symptomatic forms:
- Early myoclonic encephalopathy;
- Infant epileptic encephalopathy with areas of the isoelectric EEG;Other symptomatic generalized forms of epilepsy;
- Symptomatic generalized forms of epilepsy of specific etiology (see annex).

3. EPILEPSIA AND SYNDROME WITH UNCONDITIONAL AS FOCAL OR GENERALIZED BY ACCESSORIES

3.1. Together, generalized and focal seizures:
- Attacks of newborns;
- Severe myoclonic epilepsy of early childhood;
- Epilepsy with prolonged peak-waves on the EEG during a slow phase of sleep;
- Aphasia-epilepsy syndrome (Landau-Kleffner);
- Other vague forms of epilepsy.

3.2. Without certain generalized and focal signs (many cases of generalized tonic-clonic convulsions, which according to the clinic and EEG data can not be attributed to other forms of epilepsy of this classification, as well as many cases of large seizures during sleep).

4. SPECIAL SYNDROME

Situational (casual) seizures:
- Febrile convulsions;
- Isolated seizures or isolated status epilepticus;
- Attacks related solely to the acute effects of metabolic or toxic factors, as well as deprivation (sleep deprivation), alcohol, drugs, eclampsia, etc.

The main distinctive features of epilepsy and pseudo-epileptic seizures

Symptom	Pseudoepileptic seizures	Epilepsy
The provoking factor	Usually	May be
Признак	Pseudoepileptic seizures	Epilepsy
Start	Gradual within minutes	Sudden
Frequency	Very high	Depends on the severity of the process

Duration	Minutes and tens of minutes	Usually not > 1 minute
Аура	Trembling, faintness, emotional experience	Characteristic for localization of focus
Consciousness	Can be changed, but not lost	As a rule lost
Convulsions	Asymmetric, arrhythmic, do not correspond to topical neurophysiology	Rhythmic, symmetrical, with focalities correspond topical neurophysiology
Move	Wild movements, kolotyaschie, promiscuous, tearing, scattering, rotations, swinging with signs of production	Rhythmic symmetrical tonic convulsive-clonic myoclonic involuntary
Eye	Closed, with a passive opening stand on the line of direct vision, floating movements - coordinated	Open, wound over the supra-angled arcs, floating movements are discordant
The reaction of pupils to light	Saved	Naysayut, weakened
Vocalization	Emotional speech, more meaningful, aggressive-sensual, non-normative	Automatic machines, screams, 1 co-operative Scraps of speech
Traumatism	Rarely, insignificant	Often, sometimes heavy
Loss of urine	May be	Often
Vegetative support	Not typical	always
Emotional behavior	Обычно	Not typical
Symptoms after a fit	No	Parezy, sopor, coma, indescribable sleep
Biochemical changes	no	yes
EEG changes during an attack	No	The pattern of epileptic admission, seizure-related desynchronization
EEG changes after seizure	No	Epileptiform activity, delta activity, suppression activity
Interstitial EEG	Normally, there may be changes	Pathological and epileptiform activity

General characteristics of idiopathic generalized epilepsy

The age of the manifestation: in the majority - children's, in some - a young man and a young adult.

A picture of seizures: convulsive or non-convulsive seizures without the recognition of focalities.

EEG: Out of fit without focal changes. Generally, generalized bilateral-synchronous epileptiform activity.

During the seizure: generalized epileptiform activity without signs of locality, usually bilateral-synchronous.

Non-neurological symptoms: usually absent.

Psyche: in most cases, no features, in some cases, mental and behavioral disorders.

Neuroradiology: without structural changes.

Etiology: polygenic or multifactorial inheritance.

Prognosis: bowl-favorable, sometimes lifelong reception of drugs.

Therapy: VPA (Depakin chrono, Denikin chronosphere, Depakin-syrup), LVTSTS, LTG, TPM, FB, PWM. Not recommended KBZ. OKBZ, FT, with absences - FB.

The diagnosis of epilepsy is not made in the case of:

1. reflex (stimulus-dependent) seizures;
2. alcohol-induced seizures (with alcohol consumption or withdrawal);
3. drug-induced seizures;
4. seizures in the acute period of craniocerebral trauma (CCT);
5. A single seizure or series of seizures throughout the day, which are equated to a single fit;
6. rarely repeated seizures (oligoepilepsy).

General principles of therapy include the selection of an adequate AED corresponding to the form of epilepsy, syndrome and types of seizures. When deciding to start therapy, it is always necessary to take into account the potential danger of prolonged use of AED and related side effects.

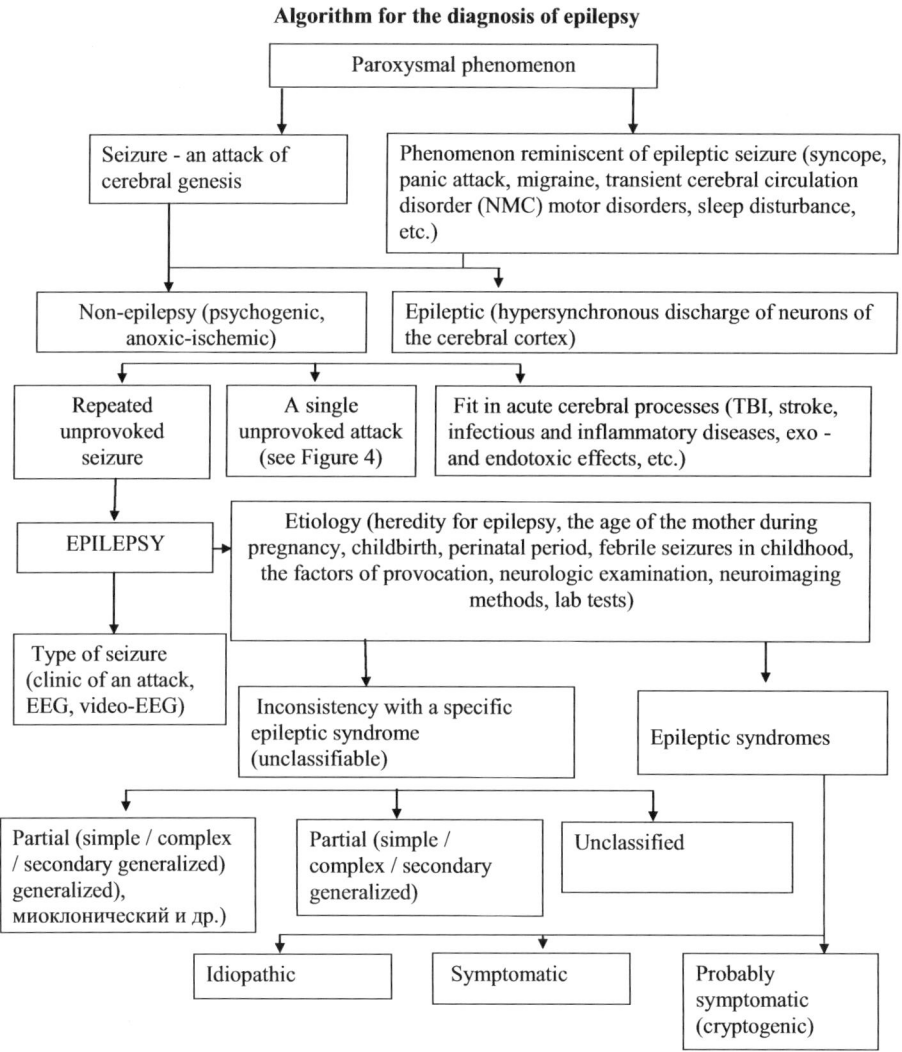

Differential-diagnostic algorithm of paroxysmal motor outbreaks

Paroxysmal locomotor disorders (according to NICT 2004 with changes)

Generalized convulsive (syncope with secondary convulsions, primary cardiac or respiratory disorders, realized in anoxic seizures, involuntary motor disorders, hyperaxple, non-epileptic attacks)

Drop-attacks (cardiovascular disorders, motor disorders, cataplexy, metabolic disorders, idiopathic drop-attacks, dyskirculation in the vertebral-basilar basin)

Transient focal motor attacks (tics, transient NCM, paroxysmal locomotor disorders, tonic spasms in multiple sclerosis)

Motor phenomena in the muscles of the face of the eyeballs (tics, facial, hemispasm, facial paraspasm)

Episodic manifestations in a dream (physiological movements, pathological fragmentary myoclonus, restless legs syndrome, REM / nonREM parasomnia, sleep apnea, other movements in a dream)

Algorithm for diagnosis and treatment of the first arising fugitive

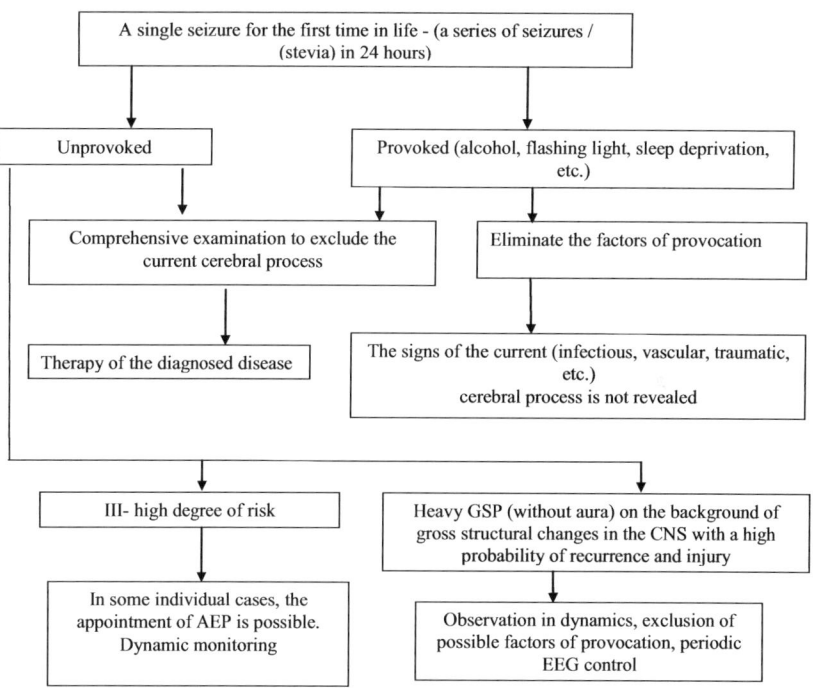

An algorithm for managing patients with epilepsy during pregnancy

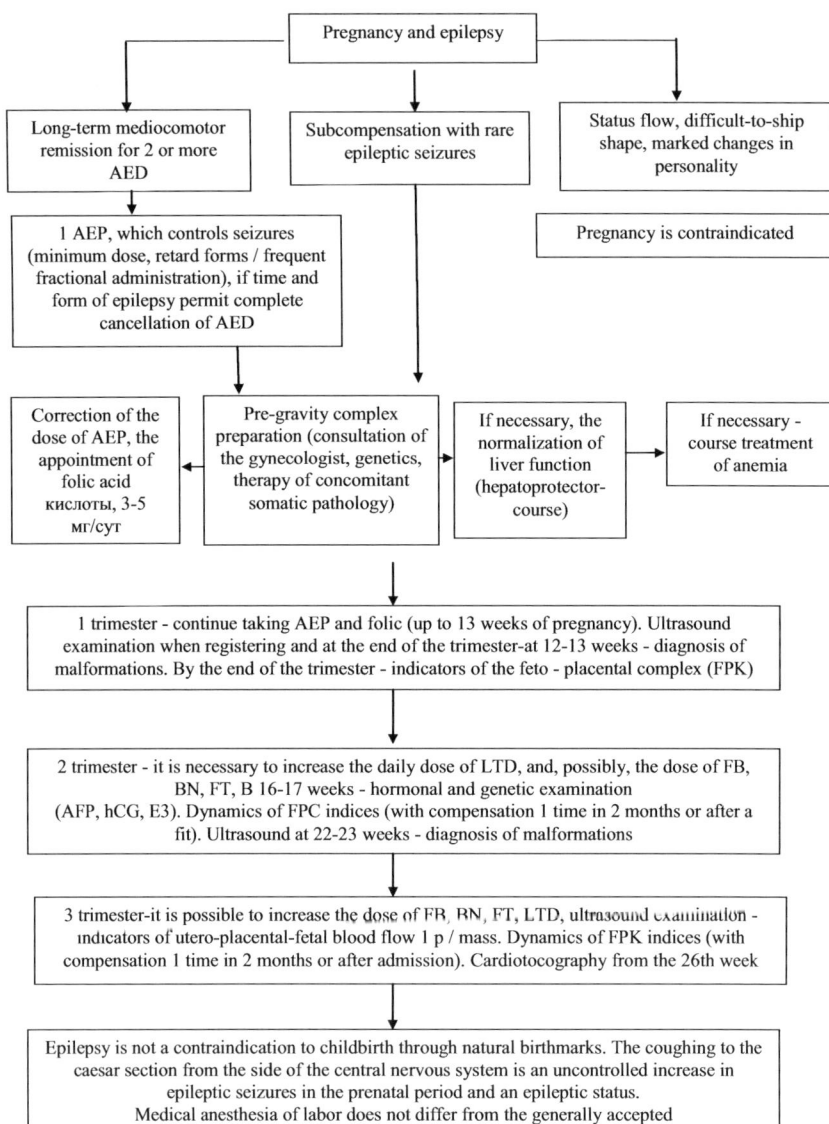

**Drugs used in the treatment of patients with various forms of epilepsy
[Schmidt D., 1996, in the modification]**

The form of epilepsy	Sequence of choice of anticonvulsants
Idiopathic partial epilepsy	Carbamazepine
	Sultiam
	Valproate sodium
	Carbamazepine
	Valproate sodium
	Phenytoin
	Vigabatrin
	Lamotrigine
	Clobazam
Symptomatic Partial Epilepsies	Valproate sodium
	Ethosuximide
	Lamotrigine
	Clobazam
	Mesuksimide
	Phenobarbital / primidon
Idiopathic generalized epilepsies: Pediatric absence epilepsy	
	Valproate sodium
Juvenile Absence Epilepsy	Lamotrigine
	Phenobarbital / primidos
	Clobazam
	Valproate sodium Phenobarbital / primidon
Juvenile myoclonic epilepsy	Clobazam
	Lamotrigine
Epilepsy with seizures of grand mal awakening	
Cryptogeic / symptomatic generalized epilepsies: Vesta Syndrome	Valproate sodium
	Vigabatrin
	ACTH, hydrocortisone
	Clobazam
Lennox-Gasto syndrome	Valproate sodium
	Lamotrigine

| | Ethosuximide
Carbamazepine
Felbamat
Clobazam |
|---|---|
| Myoclonic-astatic epilepsy | Valproate sodium
Lamotrigine
Clobazam |
| Epilepsy with myoclonic absences | Valproate sodium
Ethosuximide
Lamotrigine
Clobazam |

	Combinations of anticonvulsants
Symptomatic partial epilepsy	Carbamazepine + valproate sodium
Carbamazepine + vigabatrin
Carbamazepine + lamotrigine
Phenytoin + lamotrigine
Absence epilepsy	Valproate sodium + ethosuximide
Valproate sodium + lamotrigine
Valproate sodium + clobazam
Lennox-Gasto syndrome Myoclonic-astatic epilepsy	Valproate sodium + lamotrigine
Valproate sodium + ethosuximide
Valproate sodium + carbamazepine
Myoclonic forms of epilepsy	Valproate sodium + clobazam

Valproate sodium + lamotrigine
Valproate sodium + clobazam |

Algorithm for the treatment of focal symptomatic (cryptogenic) epilepsy

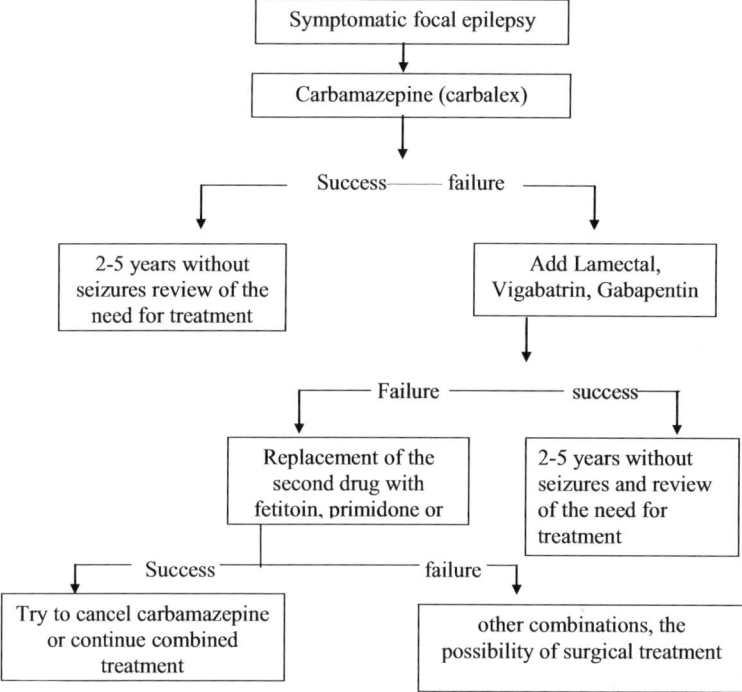

Comments:

- with the initial selection of treatment to strive for monotherapy;
- if the patient was not treated with valproate, an additional drug in combination - valproate;
- when stable remission is achieved without side effects, even on polytherapy, do not change the treatment regimen;
- general rule (with the exception of benign idiopathic forms) for partial epilepsy - treatment for at least 5 years after the last seizure; the question of cancellation of treatment earlier than this period is considered only on the initiative of the patient

Algorithm for treatment of idiopathic epilepsy with absences

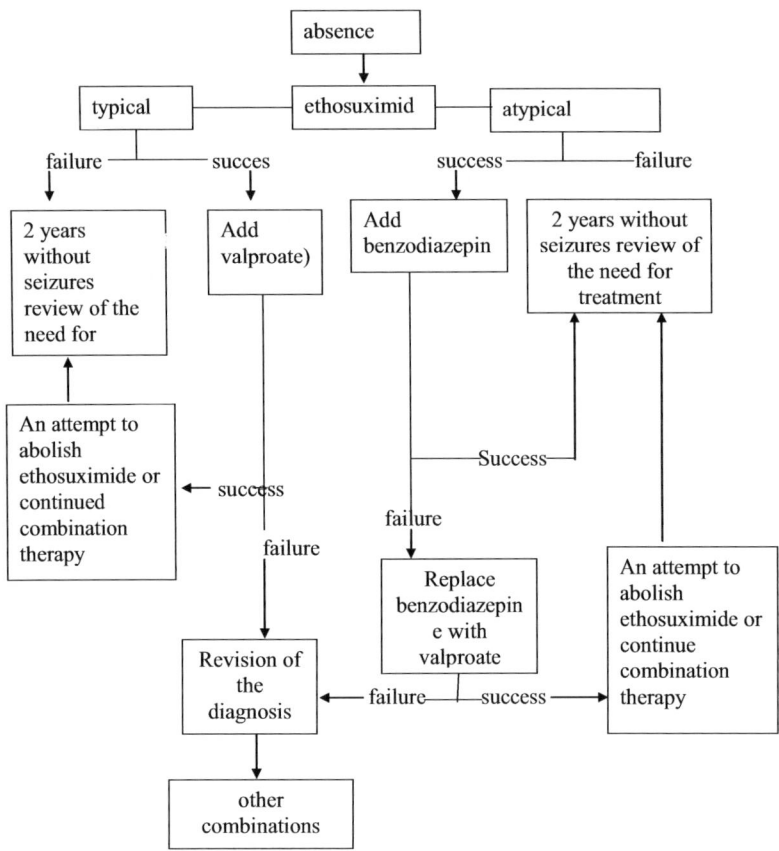

Comments:
- remember the development of tolerance to benzodiazepines and use them only as additional intermittent therapy;
- in adolescence, one should not rush with the abolition of pharmacotherapy until the completion of puberty; the question of canceled treatment is considered only on the initiative of the patient

Algorithm for treatment of idiopathic generalized epilepsy with tonic-clonic seizures

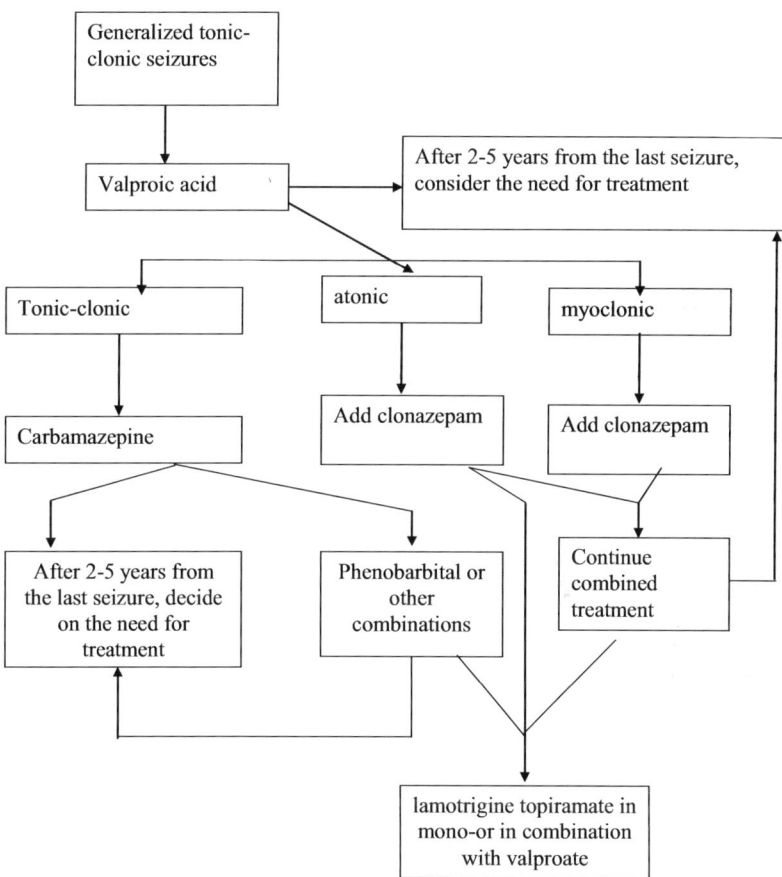

Epileptic status in adults

GENERAL PLAN OF ACTIVITIES FOR THE BUILDING OF THE EPILETIC STATUS OF TONIC AND CLONIC PAROXISMS
[DuncanJ.S. etal., 1995]

I stage (0-10 min)
Evaluation of heart and lung function
Ensuring airway patency for the purpose of aspiration prophylaxis with vomiting
Assignment of oxygen

II stage (0-60 min)
Provide monitoring of vital functions (pulse, arterial pressure, respiratory rate, ECG)
Emergency anticonvulsant therapy (diazepam, lorazepam, fe-nitooin)
The use of rapid diagnostic methods (general blood test, glucose, urea, electrolytes in blood, activity of enzymes, blood gas composition, general urine analysis)
Intravenous administration of glucose (50 ml in a 50% solution) and / or 250 mg of thiamine
Correction of metabolic acidosis (sodium bicarbonate)

III stage (0-60 / 90 min)
Carrying out the necessary diagnostic procedures (CT, MRI brain, lumbar puncture)
Identification and correction of complications

IV stage (30-90 min)
Transfer of the patient to the intensive care unit. Intensive therapy and EEG monitoring. Supportive antiepileptic therapy
Specific forms of status with mental retardation
Epileptic status in adults
- Status of absences denovo with a late debut

Transfer of the patient to the intensive care unit. Intensive therapy and EEG monitoring. Supportive antiepileptic therapy

Status stage	Preparations
Prodromal	Diazepam - 10 mg intravenously or rectally, repeated administration after 15 min
If the seizures continue: Early	First choice: *epileptic status of lorazepam - 4 mg intravenously, reintroduction* 10 min Diazepam - 10 mg intravenously, re-introduction after 15 min Second choice: Phenytoin - 250 mg (5 ml) intravenously
If the seizures continue for more than 30 minutes: Developed phenobarbitone - 10 mg / kg at a speed of epileptic status of 100 mg / min (total 600 mg per 6 min) and / or phenytoin - 18 mg / kg at a rate of 50 mg / min (1000 mg per 20 min)	
If the seizures last 60 minutes or more Resistant status epilepticus General anesthesia	

EMERGENCY ANTI-EPILOPTIC THERAPY
DEPENDING ON THE STAGE OF EPILETIC STATUS
[Cockere/l O.C., 5horvon 5.0., 1996]

Status stage	Preparations

Prodromal

Diazepam - 10 mg intravenously or rectally, repeated administration after 15 min

If the seizures continue:

Early:
First choice:
The epileptic status of Lorazepam is 4 mg intravenously, repeated administration after 10 minutes.
Diazepam - 10 mg intravenously, repeated administration after 15 min
Second choice:

Phenytoin - 250 mg (5 ml) intravenously **If the seizures continue for more than 30 minutes:**
Developed:
- **Phenobarbitone** 10 mg / kg at speed
- epileptic status of 100 mg / min (total 600 mg per 6 min) and / or
- Phenytoin - 18 mg / kg at a rate of 50 mg / min (1000 mg per 20 min)
If the seizures last 60 minutes or more:
Resistant   General Anesthesia
status epilepticus

MOISTENIES, MIASTENIC CRISES

Myasthenia gravis is a disease caused by a violation of neuromuscular transmission due to a decrease in the number of cholinergic receptors of the terminal plate of synapses and (or) their insufficient sensitivity to acetylcholine.

Myasthenia gravis acquired congenital (genetically-determined) neonatal.

The pathogenetic mechanism is an autoimmune process. Changes in the thymus gland (hyperplasia or hyperfunction without increase) lead to the production of antibodies to the protein of the cholinergic receptors to the striated muscles. Autoantibodies bind to the protein of acetylcholine receptors, cause degradation and destroy gradually the membrane, as a result of which the synaptic cleft dilates, the possibility of impulse is reduced, since acetylcholine enters but does not bind or bind to a small number of receptors.

Classification

I. By age of origin:
1. Neonatal. May be in children from mothers suffering from myasthenia gravis or transient myasthenia gravis of newborns (sluggish child syndrome).
2. Myasthenia gravis.
3. Myasthenia gravis of adults.

II. By detecting antibodies:
1. seropositive
2. seronegative.

III. Clinical classification of myasthenia gravis (BM Hecht in 1965):

1. The nature of the course of the myasthenic process:
- myasthenic episode,
- myasthenic state,
- Progressive myasthenia gravis,
- malignant myasthenia gravis;

2. Degree of generalization of motor disorders:
- local processes (eye, bulbar, facial, cranial, trunk forms);
- generalized:
a) without disturbance of breathing, b) with respiratory failure;
3. Severity of motor disorders:
- Light;
- Average;
- heavy;

4. Degree of motor impairment compensation: complete;
- sufficient (for self-service in the home); - плохая (нуждается в постороннем уходе

By degree of hyperplasia:
a) generalized
b) local

On the degree of motor disorders:
a) easy
b) mean
c) heavy.

On the intensity of recovery of motor function after the introduction of AHEP (degree of compensation):
a) complete
b) incomplete
c) bad.

The presence of violations of vital functions.
Diagnostics
The striated muscles are more often affected:
• oculomotor (60-90%)

- Facial (75%)
- Chewing (30%)
- Bulbar (30%)
- Muscles of the extremities of the hand (77%), legs (55%)
- Muscles of the neck and trunk (30%).
1. Based on clinical manifestations (myasthenic syndrome).
2. Electrophysiological study (ENMG).
3. Serological.

Clinical Trials:
1. Proserin test - enter
Sol.Proserini 0.05% 1-3 ml / k +
Sol.Atropini 0.1% - 0.5 ml
Evaluation after 30 minutes. For example, reduction of ptosis, restoration of articulation during reading, etc.
2. Electrophysiological. ENMG - decrease in the amplitude of the action potential min by 10% of the norm. Better 12-15% with stimulating ENMG.
3. Serological determination of the level of antibodies to choline receptors and striated muscles in the blood.
4. X-ray computed tomography or magnetic resonance imaging of mediastinal organs. Reliability in detecting thymoma is 95%.

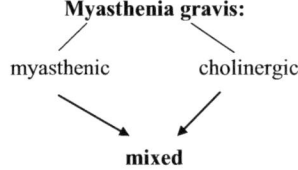

	MIASTENIC CRISES
FACTORS. DEVELOPING METHODS	- Instability of breathing and bulbar symptoms; - Elderly and old age; - Chronic and intercurrent somatic diseases; - The presence of thymoma; - Early emerging myasthenic crises; - Female gender)
MEDICINES, PROMOTING	A / 6 preparations: aminoglycosides, tetracyclines,

THE DEVELOPMENT OF MK	sulfamides, ciprofloxacin; - Antiepileptic drugs: barbiturates, carbamazepine, diphenin; - Psychotropic drugs: aminazine, lithium preparations, tricyclic antidepressants, amitriptyline; - Hormonal preparations: ACTH, OK, oxytocin, thyroid hormones; - Cardiological agents: ß-blockers, lidocaine, novocaine, calcium ion antagonists, ganglion blockers; - Other drugs: morphine derivatives, muscle relaxants, radiopaque substances.
SAFE PREPARATIONS	- A / 6 preparations: cephalosporins of III and IV generations, levomitsetin, rifampicin, isoniazid, nitrofurans; - Antiepileptic drugs: lamotrigine, valproate; - Psychotropic drugs: sanopax, benzodiazepines in small doses; - Cardiological agents: digoxin, methyldopa, spirorolactone, triamtrene; - Analgesics and anti-inflammatory drugs: NSAIDs, paracetamol, diclofenac
FACTORS, PROVIDING THE DEVELOPMENT OF MK	Bacterial or viral infection of the VAP; Decompaction of diabetes mellitus; - Severe dehydration, which breaks VEB; - Surgical operations conducted under anesthesia; Stopping the intake of glucocorticoid hormones or immunosuppressive drugs.
SYMPTOMS DECOMPOSATION OF THE MOISTENCE	Sharp, rapid weight loss; - Increasing demand for AChE preparations; - Increasing difficulty in swallowing, chewing and coughing; -Increased weakness of the neck muscles ("hanging head"); - Difficulty in breathing due to weakness of the diaphragm and pectoral muscles.

Differential-diagnostic criteria for crises

Symptoms	Myasthenic crisis	Cholinergic crisis
The size of pupils	Wide	Narrow, paresis of accommodation
Arterial pressure	Tachycardia	Bradycardia
Arterial pressure	Normal or Slightly Reduced	A sharp decline
Muscular fascination	Not typical	Strongly expressed
Abdominal pain, violent intestinal peristalsis, vomiting, diarrhea	Not typical	Strongly expressed
Shortness of breath, aphonia, impossible to expectorate	Very characteristic	Not typical

Treatment of myasthenia gravis

It is aimed at correcting the relative deficiency of acetylcholine and inhibiting the autoimmune process. In order to compensate for the disorders neuromuscular transmission using anticholinesterase drugs: proserine, oxazil, kalimin. It is important to choose the optimal individually compensating dose depending on the clinical form, the severity of the symptoms, the concomitant diseases, the reaction to the drug. With glandular and ocular forms of myasthenia gravis, pyridostigmine bromide is more effective, with myasthenic weakness of skeletal musculature - proserine and oxazyl. Doses of drugs and intervals of admission are individual. Assign chloride or potassium orotate, veroshpiron, ephedrine. In very severe cases, parenterally injected proserin (1.5-2 ml of 0.05% solution intramuscularly) for 20-30 minutes before meals. Taking large doses of anticholinesterase drugs can lead to a cholinergic crisis. The main method of treatment of this crisis is the abolition of anticholinergics and the repeated administration of atropine (0.5 ml 0.1% solution intravenously or subcutaneously). In severe cases, you can appoint a cholinesterase reagent (1 ml of a 15% solution of dipyroxime).

When the myasthenic crisis occurs as a result of an insufficient dose of anticholinesterase drugs, intravenous intravenous (0.5-1 ml 0.05% solution) and intramuscularly (2-3 ml after 2-3 hours) are urgently injected. Oxazyl can be administered in candles. Apply also a 5% solution of ephedrine subcutaneously, potassium preparations intravenously. The progressive and life-threatening weakness of the respiratory muscles can be observed despite the introduction of large quantities of proserin. Patients undergo intubation or tracheostomy, and are transferred to mechanical ventilation using breathing apparatus. Nutrition of patients is carried out through a nasogastric tube. It is necessary to maintain a balance of liquid and electrolytes, vitamins; According to the indications (metabolic acidosis), 1% solution of sodium hydrogencarbonate is injected intravenously.

The main methods of pathogenetic treatment of myasthenia gravis patients are thymectomy, X-ray therapy and hormone therapy. The surgical method (thymectomy) is indicated to all patients under the age of 60 suffering from myasthenia gravis, but in a satisfactory condition. It is absolutely indicated for tumors of the thymus gland. X-ray therapy on the area of this gland is prescribed with the remainder of its tissue after thymectomy, with the myasthenia eye form, and also in the presence of contraindications to surgery in elderly patients with a generalized form of myasthenia gravis. In severe cases - with generalized myasthenia gravis - treatment with immunosuppressive drugs is indicated. Assign corticosteroids, the best prednisolone (100 mg every other day). The duration of taking the maximum dose of corticosteroids is limited by the onset of a significant improvement, which subsequently allows the dose to be reduced to a supporting dose.

Plasmapheresis and intravenous immunoglobulin are used to relieve exacerbations and myasthenic crisis. Plasmapheresis is also performed with preoperative preparation of patients. The optimal scheme is the replacement of 2-3 liters of plasma 3 times a week (a total of 5-6 sessions). According to foreign studies, more effective daily procedures, however it is connected with the big risk of disturbance of a water-electrolyte balance, disorders of a hemostasis and a hypoalbuminemia. Immunoglobulin is administered intravenously for 2-5 days in a total dose of 2 g per 1 kg of body weight. The method is effective in 78% of patients

Auxiliary therapy includes metabolic therapy: antioxidants, vitamins B, E, D, anabolics - are better non-steroid, as more often women are ill, such as riboxin, ATP. The use of retabolil in women is undesirable. Retabolil 5% solution 1 ml in / m №6 after 3 days, then 1 ml after 5-7-10-12-20-30 days, then maintain a dose of 1 ml IM in 2 months.

Treatment of crises.

1. As the first event, the need for adequate breathing with the help of forced ventilation. According to the indications for the transfer to artificial ventilation - a violation of the rhythm of breathing, cyanosis, agitation, loss of consciousness, participation of auxiliary muscles, changes in pupil size, no response to the administration of AChE preparations.

2. Conduction of plasmapheresis or plasmosorption. It is carried out by a course for 1-2 weeks with a multiplicity of 2-5 operations.

3. Immunoglobulins. Human Ig is an immunoreactive protein. The drugs are excreted from the plasma of healthy people. The use of high doses of Ig has the ability to suppress immune processes. Currently, Ig therapy is an alternative to plasmapheresis, based on the similarities of the mechanisms underlying these treatments.

A common treatment regimen is a short 5-day course of IV administration of the drug at a dose of 400 mg / kg daily. On the average, the clinical effect is observed on day 4 of therapy and lasts for 50-100 days. Experience can also be used with the introduction of minimum doses of octagam and bioven 4-5 mg / kg iv drip No.10, the total dose of 25 grams.

The possibility of using normal human Ig in a dose of 50 ml is drip by 100-150 ml of physiological solution. Introductions are repeated every other day in the amount of 3-5 grams per course of treatment.

4. Anticholinesterase drugs. Parenteral administration is most often used. Prozerin is administered sc 1.5 to 2.5 ml, atropine 0.2-0.5 ml of a 01% solution is administered to reduce unwanted effects. The result is estimated as in the proserin test.

5. Glucocorticosteroid preparations. The most effective application of pulse therapy is 1000 mg of methylprednisolone intravenously. After that, it is recommended to use daily Prednisolone.

BIBLIOGRAPHY

1. Akimov G.A. Initial manifestations of cerebral vascular diseases: Medical Sciences, 1983, 209 p.
2. Akimov GA, Erokhina LG Neurology of syncopal states. - M., 1987, 208 p.
3. Antonov I.N., Shanko G.G. Hyperkinesis in children. - Minsk, 1975,216 pages.
4. Badalyan L.O. Pediatric Neurology. M .: Medicine, 2001, 416 pp.
5. Baranshev Yu.I. Perinatal neurology. Publishing house "Triad X", Moscow, 2001. 640p.
6. Bogolepov NK, Mikheev VV Vascular diseases of the nervous system and diseases of the autonomic nervous system. In the book: a multivolume guide to neurology. T. IV Medgiz-1963,342 p.
7. Wein A.M. Vegetative disorders. Clinic, diagnosis, treatment. M .: Medicine, 1998, 752 p.
8. Wayne AM Pain syndromes in neurological practice. Moscow, Medpress, 1999, 364 pages.
9. Viderkholst VK Treatment of Nervous Diseases, Medicine, Moscow, 1994, 536 p.
10. Voloshin P.V., Taitslin V.I. Treatment of vascular diseases of the brain and spinal cord. "Knowledge-M" "Knowledge" Zaporozhye 1999.553.
11. Vorlow ChP, Denis MS, Van J. Heine, G.Zh. Khankiy and others. Stroke. Practical guidance for managing patients. Polytechnic. Publishing house St. Petersburg 1998, 614 p.
12. Gusev EI, Burd GS, Nikiforov AS Neurological symptoms, syndromes, symptom-complexes and diseases. Moscow, Medicine, 1999, 824 pages.
13. Guzeva V.I. A guide to children's neurology. St. Petersburg, 1998, 495s.
14. Gusev EI, Yakhno NN, Sanadze AG, Mechanisms of development and principles of treatment of diseases of the peripheral nervous system, Moscow, 2007, 234 p.
15. Gusev EI, Skvortsova V.I. Ischemia of the brain. M .: Medicine, 2001, 326 p.
16. Gusev EI, Konovalov AN, Burd GS Neurology and Neurosurgery. Moscow: Medicine, 2000, 240 pages.
17. Guzeva VI, Mikhailov IB, Pharmacotherapy of nerve diseases in adults and children. Moscow: Medicine, 2002, 400 p.
18. Golubev VL Selected lectures on neurology. "Eidos Media", Moscow, 2004, 624 pages.

19. David O. Vibers, Valery Feigin, Robert D. Brown. Manual on cerebrovascular diseases, Moscow 1999, 240 pp.

20. Duschanova G.A. Neurology. 1.2 part. 2000. 276 p.

21. Zharkov PL. Osteochondrosis and other dystrophic changes in the dystrophic changes in the spine in adults and children. M.: Medicine, 1994. 376 p.

22. Zavalishin NA, Golovkina V.I. Multiple sclerosis. Moscow, 2000. 640s.

23. Zenkov LR, Ronkin MA Functional diagnostics of nerve diseases M .: Medicine, 1991, 240 pages.

24. Zenkov, L.R. Treatment of epilepsy. Moscow, 2001, 220p.

25. Zenkov LR Modern treatment of epilepsy. A Guide for Physicians, Moscow, 2001, 129 pp.

26. Kaishibaev S.K. Neurology. I, 2 part. Almaty, 1998, 298 pages

27. V.V. Karlov. Neurology. Moscow: Medicine, 2002, 236 pages.

28. Konovalov A. N. Neurotraumatology. The book "Vasar-Ferro" Moscow, 1997, 411 pages.

29. V.V. Karlov. Therapy of nervous diseases. M .: Medicine, 1995, 512 pages.

30. Kirpichenko AA and others. Nervous and mental illnesses. Minsk, 1997, 367 pages.

31. Clinical protocols of management and treatment of patients with acute stroke. They are confirmed by the protocol of the Expert Council of the Ministry of Health of the Republic of Kazakhstan. of April 17, 2012 No. 8

32. Konovalov AN, Likhterman LB, Potapov AA Clinical Manual for Cerebral Trauma. - M .: "Antidor", 1998. - v.1.2.630 p.

33. Lebedev B.V. Spravochnik on Neurology of Childhood M .: Medicine, 1995, 576 p.

34. Mukhin K. Yu., Petrukhin AS, Idiopathic forms of epilepsy: systematics, diagnostics, therapy. "Art-Business Center" Moscow, 2000, 319 pages.

35. Martynov Yu.S. Nervous diseases. M .: Medicine, 1999, 123 p.

36. Mikhailenko AA Clinical Workshop on Neurology. S.Peterburg, 2001, 480 p.

37. Odinak M.M. Topical diagnosis of diseases and injuries of the nervous system. St. Petersburg, 1997, 232 pp.

38. Pepelyansky Y.Yu. Diseases of the peripheral nervous system. M .: Medicine, 1989., 463 p.

39. Peter Duus Topical diagnosis in neurology. Moscow, "Vasar-Ferro", 1996, 378 pages.

40. Sarah Hexil, Arthur Merlyan. Pediatric Neurology and Neurosurgery M: Medicine, 1996., 236 p.

41. Skoromets AA, Thyssen TP, Panyushkin AI, Skoromets TA Vascular diseases of the spinal cord. Sotis St. Petersburg 1998. 481 p.

42. Samoylov VI Syndromological diagnosis of diseases of the nervous system. IPC "Biant" Saint-Petersburg, 1998, 411 pages.

43. Temina P.A., Nikanorova M.Yu. Epilepsy and convulsive syndromes in children: A guide for doctors / Under red.-2-ed., Pererab. and additional .- M .: Medicine, 1999.- 656 p.

44. Triumphov A.V. Topical diagnosis of diseases of the nervous system. L.: Medicine, 1996, 264 pages.

45. Troshin VM, Burtsev EM, Troshin V.D. Angioneurology of childhood M. 1995, 480 pp.

46. Umansky K.G. Neurology for all. M .: Medicine, 1995, 317 pages.

47. Farber MA, Farber FM Neuropathies of the facial nerve. Almaty, 2004, 217 pages.

48. Fedin AI, Rumyantseva SA Intensive therapy of ischemic stroke. A guide for doctors. Moscow, 2004, 280 pp.

49. Farber MA, Majidov NM Lumbar osteochondrosis and its neurologic syndromes. Tashkent, 1996, 211 pages.

50. Hertl M. Differential diagnosis in pediatrics. In 2 volumes. M: Medicine, 1990, 511 pages.

51. Khodos BG Nervous diseases. A guide for doctors. Moscow: Medicine, 2001, 512 pages.

52. Shtulman, DR, Levin, OS Neurology. Medpress-Inform, 2007, 935 pages.

53. Shmidt IR Vertebrogenic syndrome of the vertebral artery. Novosibirsk, Publisher, 2001, 271 pages.

54. Shamansurov Sh.Sh., Troshin VM, Kravtsov Yu.I. Pediatric Neurology. Publishing house of med.it.im.Ablu Ali ibn Sino, 1995, 648 p.

55. Shabalov NP, Yaroslavsky VK, Khodov DA, Lyubimenko VA Asphyxia of newborns. L .: Medicine, 1990, 368 pages.

56. Shtok V.N. Pharmacotherapy in neurology. M .: Medicine, 2006, 477p.

57. Yakhno N.N., Shtulman D.A. Nervous diseases. I and II volume. M .: Medicine, 2001, 1256 p.

58. Yakhno NN, Damulin I.V. Encephalopathy. / Methodological recommendations

Content

1. Introduction 3
2. Diseases of the peripheral nervous system 4
3. Conditional Symbols and Abbreviations...........................…..7
4. Cervical Irritative Reflex Syndroms…………………………. 9
5. Infectious diseases of the nervous system 49
6. Craniocerebral injury. Classification 88
7. Vascular diseases of the nervous system 99
8. Epilepsy 150
9. Myasthenia gravis, myasthenic crises……………….....…..….168
10. Bibliography.. 173
11. Content……………………………………………………..… 176

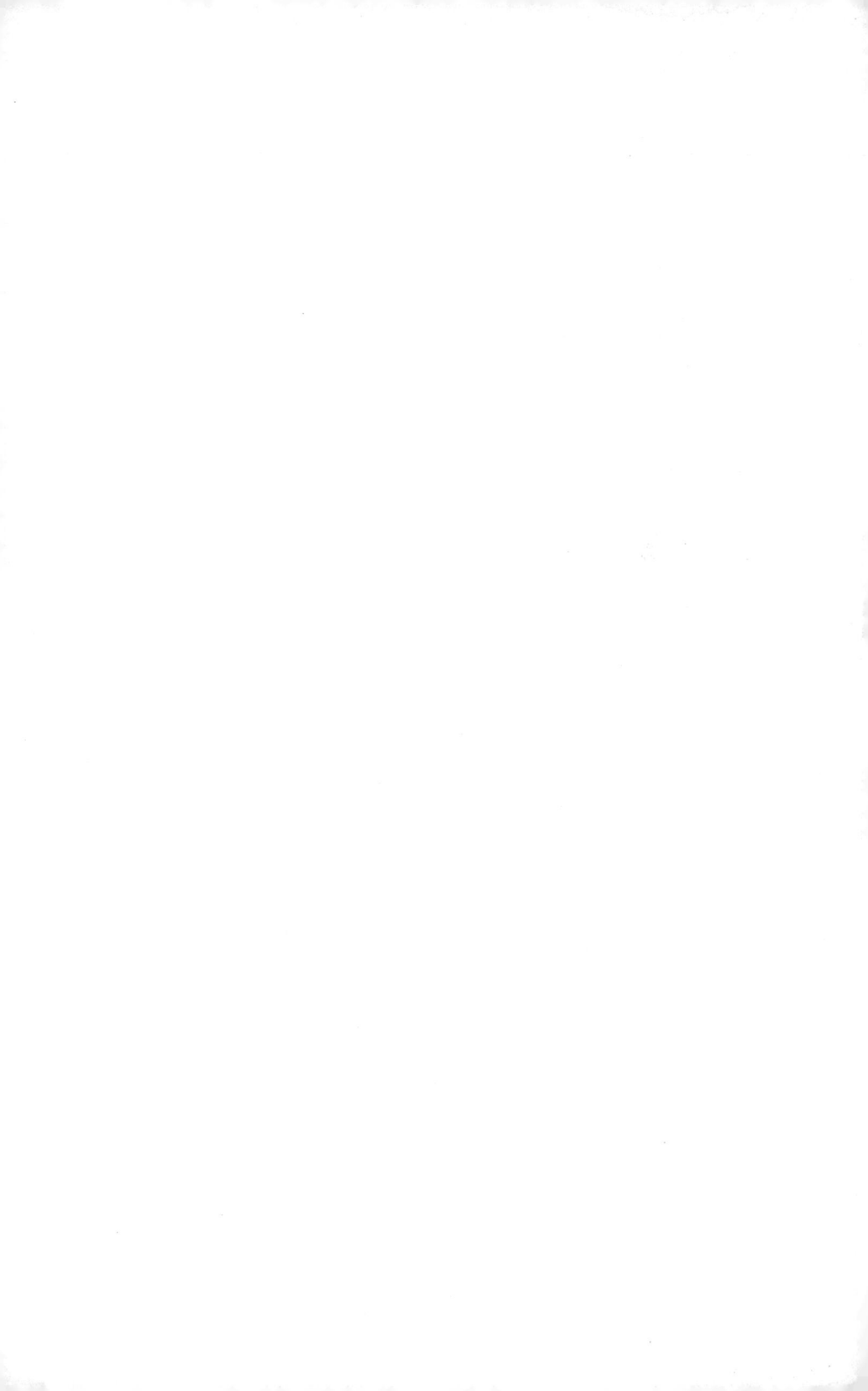

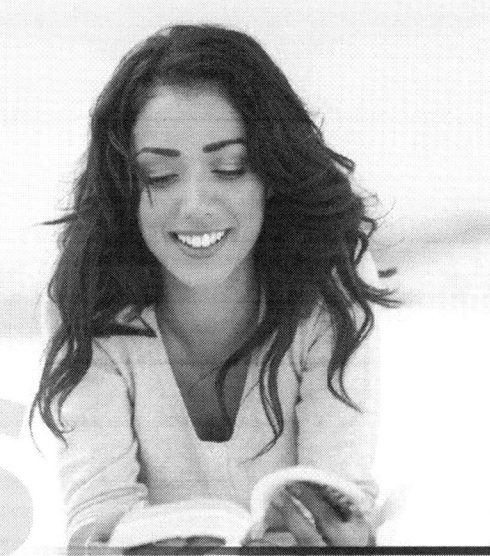

I want morebooks!

Buy your books fast and straightforward online - at one of the world's fastest growing online book stores! Environmentally sound due to Print-on-Demand technologies.

Buy your books online at
www.get-morebooks.com

Kaufen Sie Ihre Bücher schnell und unkompliziert online – auf einer der am schnellsten wachsenden Buchhandelsplattformen weltweit! Dank Print-On-Demand umwelt- und ressourcenschonend produziert.

Bücher schneller online kaufen
www.morebooks.de

SIA OmniScriptum Publishing
Brivibas gatve 1 97
LV-103 9 Riga, Latvia
Telefax: +371 68620455

info@omniscriptum.com
www.omniscriptum.com

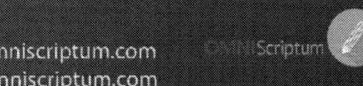

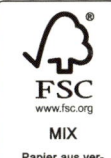

Druck:
Customized Business Services GmbH
im Auftrag der
KNV Zeitfracht GmbH
Ein Unternehmen der Zeitfracht - Gruppe
Ferdinand-Jühlke-Str. 7
99095 Erfurt